# The
# M
# Workbook

...The majority of candidates [who fail the MRCGP] give the impression that reading is so far down their list of priorities as to be virtually out of sight. It is not so much a question of lack of relevant/appropriate reading, or inability to critically evaluate appropriate articles, but rather total absence of any reading whatsoever.

Andrew Belton
Former Chief Examiner
Royal College of General Practitioners

*For Churchill Livingstone*
*Publisher:* Lucy Gardner
*Copy Editor:* Kathryn Whyman
*Design:* Design Resources Unit and Charles Simpson
*Cover design: Keith Kail*
*Production:* Mark Sanderson
*Sales Promotion Executive:* Marion Pollock

# The MRCGP Workbook

**Neal Maskrey**
MB ChB DRCOG FRCGP

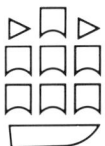

CHURCHILL LIVINGSTONE
EDINBURGH LONDON MADRID MELBOURNE NEW YORK AND TOKYO 1994

CHURCHILL LIVINGSTONE
Medical Division of Longman Group UK Limited

Distributed in the United States of America by Churchill Livingstone Inc.,
650 Avenue of the Americas, New York, N.Y. 10011, and by associated
companies, branches and representatives throughout the world.

First published 1994

ISBN 0-443-04985-8

**British Library Cataloguing in Publication Data**
A catalogue record for this book is available from the British Library.

**Library of Congress Cataloging in Publication Data**
A catalog record for this book is available from the Library of Congress.

The
publisher's
policy is to use
paper manufactured
from sustainable forests

Produced by Longman Singapore Publishers Pte Ltd.
Printed in Singapore

# Contents

Preface   vii
Acknowledgements   ix

**The MRCGP examination   1**
Aims and objectives, format and content   1
Why do candidates fail the examination?   3

**Revision programme   7**
Time available   7
Resources   8
Revision curriculum   8

**The multiple choice question paper   13**
Format   13
Content   13
Technique   14
Multiple choice question paper I   17
Multiple choice answers paper I   21
Multiple choice question paper II   23
Multiple choice answers paper II   27

**The modified essay question paper   29**
Format   29
Content   29
Practical points on technique   30
Skeletons   32
Modified essay question paper   35
Modified essay question model
    answers   47

**Critical reading question paper   59**
Format   59
Content   60
Technique   62
Critical reading question paper   63
Critical reading question model
    answers   73

**Revision topics and relevant papers   83**
Screening the elderly   83
Out-of-hours calls   86
GP obstetrics   87
Work patterns in general practice   89
Prevention   93
Alcohol   97

Computers   97
Diabetes   99
The NHS reforms   101
Audit   105
Minor illness in general practice   106
Breast cancer screening   108
Child health surveillance   109
Practice formularies   110
Asthma   110
The health of doctors   112
The menopause – hormone replacement
    therapy   113
Complementary medicine   114
Public health   115
Chronic fatigue syndrome   116
Hypertension   117
Management of myocardial infarction   120
Lipids   122
Cardiology   123
Cervical cytology   126
Miscellany   128

**The orals   131**
Format   131
Content   132
Technique   133
Oral questions   136

**Appendix   145**

# Preface

There are a number of excellent published works concerned with the content and techniques required in the membership examination of the Royal College of General Practitioners (MRCGP). In addition there is a vast amount of relevant written material recording British general practice. No one could expect to be conversant with it all but a widespread criticism of candidates who perform poorly in the MRCGP is their lack of familiarity with even a basic knowledge of the appropriate books and journals. Some appreciation of current areas of debate or controversy and the ability to evaluate and apply these issues to general practice is also required.

For some time the examiners have been looking for candidates to show this aspect of their knowledge in the oral examinations. In addition, in the autumn of 1990 the Practice Topic Question paper was replaced in the written papers by the Critical Reading Question Paper. With a 2-hour written paper devoted to assessing these attributes, a major aspect of preparing for the examination must be to become familiar with a reasonable sample of the literature of general practice.

Having organised preparation courses for the examination it is clear to me that candidates do have considerable problems in fulfilling this requirement. Not only is it hard to find the time and motivation to study whilst in most cases fulfilling a full-time service commitment, but the vast range of material to digest seems sometimes so overwhelming that it is difficult to know where to start. Furthermore, though the existing examination preparation books all carry a small bibliography, for the most part they refer to textbooks. Clearly there is a need for a guide which gives some signposts into the literature of general practice, help with examination content and technique as well as assistance with revision planning. Having received many encouraging comments on this course workbook it is to be hoped that a wider audience will now find it as useful.

The problem with any book of this nature is that with one scientific paper being published in English every 6 seconds the author and publishers will inevitably be overtaken by the contemporary medical journals. The advice to candidates from the RCGP is that reading the last 2 years' of the British Medical Journal (BMJ) and the British Journal of General Practice (BJGP) is mandatory preparation for the Critical Reading Paper. It is to be hoped that readers will find in this book a starting point in the literature from which to explore further and will continue with this educational voyage of discovery throughout the rest of their careers.

Finally, the precis that has been added below most of the papers is there only to refresh the memory of jaded examination candidates and is not an appropriate substitute for reading the original article.

N.M.

# Acknowledgements

The author and publishers gratefully acknowledge the help and cooperation of the Royal College of General Practitioners in allowing reproduction of examination material.

I would like to acknowledge the help of friends and colleagues in the preparation of this book. Amongst those who have contributed with inspiration or perspiration or both are:

Mark Williams, Andrew Belton, Walter Anderson, John Bibby, Jenny Lund, Alan Pollock, Mary Evans, Seth Jenkinson, Malcolm Stuart, the late Professor David Triger and many fellows and members of the Yorkshire Faculty of the Royal College of General Practitioners. Their help and support is greatly appreciated.

My wife Jill and daughters Alison, Elisabeth and Sarah have tolerated my disappearances into the study nobly and without their support this book would not have been completed.

Lucy Gardner at Churchill Livingstone has borne the idiosyncracies of a first-time author with cheerful fortitude. Thank you.

Neal Maskrey          Scarborough, June, 1993

# 1

# The MRCGP Examination

- Aims and objectives, format and content
- Why do candidates fail the examination?

## Aims and objectives, format and content

The College of General Practitioners was founded in November 1952. Membership was attained for the first 12 years based upon an application supported by sponsors and a personal report. Applications were open only to those who had been qualified for a minimum of 7 years and had spent at least 5 years as general practitioners.

The first examination for membership of the Royal College of General Practitioners (MRCGP) was held in March 1965. There were five candidates and all were successful. Other Royal Colleges were helpful in the early days of the examination and collaborated enthusiastically with novice GP examiners. The excellent spirit of the venture is exemplified by the report from a joint conference in 1968, a notable feature of which was that all present, including the presidents of the Royal Colleges, completed a multiple choice question paper which was marked on the day. Diplomatically this was returned without comment to the 'candidates'.

From these humble beginnings has emerged an organisation that is now responsible for one of the largest postgraduate medical examinations in the world with almost 2000 candidates each year. The RCGP examiners are highly regarded in academic circles for their expertise in this form of assessment, expertise that has steadily been refined over the years. The aims and format have been modified from time to time and will no doubt continue to alter in the future.

The numbers of candidates increased over the years until a reasonably steady state was reached in the late 1980s. The pass rate in the examination has stabilised following the increasing professional approach to making the examination reliable and valid which began in the mid 1980s, together with the production of the examiner's attributes at around the same time. The term validity refers to the extent to which a test measures what the examiners want it to measure. Reliability refers to the consistency and accuracy of the test.

Even some of the examination's sternest critics are prepared to agree that enormous efforts are made by the panel of examiners and their educational advisers to compile a fair test. It is often said that the content of the examination really does reflect the ordinary, everyday work of a general practitioner. A qualification to this is the inclusion of the occasional question that perhaps only the above average or even exceptional candidates are able to respond to appropriately.

One problem for the examiners and candidates is the endlessly expanding range of knowledge, skills and attitudes that one might be expected to possess as a GP. However, by and large the examination stays true to its roots and even unsuccessful candidates are rarely able to argue convincingly that they were asked unreasonable questions. They may have been asked *difficult* questions but if candidates were only asked questions to which they knew the answers how could examiners discover the limit of each candidate's knowledge?

The examination consists of three elements:

---

1. **Pre-certification in**
   (i) Cardiopulmonary resuscitation.
   (ii) Child health surveillance.

2. **The written papers**
   (i) Multiple Choice Question paper (MCQ)
   (ii) Modified Essay Question paper (MEQ)
   (iii) Critical Reading Question paper (CRQ).

3. **The oral examinations**
   (i) The Practice Experience Questionnaire viva.
   (ii) The Problem Solving viva.

---

This structure has changed many times over the years. Sometimes this has been in order to highlight the importance of one or other area of practice in response to the need to rectify deficiencies in the knowledge or approaches of a large number of candidates. On other occasions a change has been instituted to improve the validity or reliability of the examination. Appreciating this may help candidates understand the examiners' agenda.

Pre-certification in resuscitation skills was introduced in May 1990 following the publication of studies demonstrating the poor performance of doctors in these basic skills. The candidate is required to organise a personal assessment of resuscitation skills by an ambulance training officer, a member of St John or the Red Cross, a hospital consultant or a general practitioner who would normally undertake such training and assessment. The process usually requires a session of training, retraining or revision followed by the assessment. Often this is performed using a modern manikin which has electronic interactive teaching facilities which are able to assess the effectiveness of the resuscitation techniques being performed. The test certificate, together with the manikin performance record (if available), is returned to the examination board.

Child Health Surveillance (CHS) became applicable following the introduction of the 1990 GP contract. The College contended that the examination had always examined candidates in this area of general practice. However, the requirement of Family Health Service Authorities to create a list of GPs with the requisite skills meant that the testing needed to be beyond dispute. The pre-certification certificate is obtained from any GP principal on an FHSA's CHS list. Once again the testing may follow training or practical revision sessions.

Details of the written and oral sections are contained in later chapters.

Candidates will naturally wonder about the standard required to pass the MRCGP examination. The surprising answer is that it is theoretically possible for the standards to vary with each cohort of the examination. This is because the examination, like the huge majority of British undergraduate and postgraduate medical examinations, is a norm referenced test rather than a criterion referenced test.

An example of a criterion referenced test is the British driving test. Providing we do our three point turn, emergency stop, park correctly, know our highway code and generally proceed in a safe driving manner we will pass the test. In any given month it could be that no one achieves the required standard or that everyone achieves it. The pass *rate* may therefore vary but the pass *mark* is predetermined.

In a norm referenced test the scores achieved by candidates are ranked on a normal distribution curve and the pass mark is adjusted to a predetermined pass/failure rate. This means that it is theoretically possible for a candidate to be very lucky and sit the examination with a cohort who perform below average and pass, whereas on another occasion, with an exceptionally able cohort, the same candidate might fail. It would even be possible for a candidate with sufficient private means to pay 100 doctors to sit the written papers and get them to significantly under-perform, thus artificially moving the genuine candidates up the normal distribution curve. One could think of better ways of spending £30 000 but it is possible.

It is extremely difficult to construct a criterion referenced medical examination. A driving test is looking at specific manual skills whereas the skills required by a general practitioner are complex and multiple, involving knowledge, skills and attitudes. They are often difficult to measure other than by inference, particularly when there are nearly 2000 candidates to be tested.

In fact the examination team goes to considerable lengths to ensure the validity and reliability of the examination. Candidates can be reassured that the MRCGP examination is, as far as is humanly possible, a fair test of the agenda which the examiners set. In reality it is safe to assume that a candidate passing or failing on one occasion would obtain the same result if sitting the examination with a different cohort. Those who fail need to do more work and rectify their technique in order to perform better on a second occasion.

The panel of examiners continues to look at the examination and its development. Currently it is looking hard at the persisting absence from the examination of any direct assessment of candidates' clinical skills. It is likely that this possible defect will be rectified in the near future by the addition of one of the following:

- a video tape of surgery consultations to be viewed as part of the examination
- candidates sitting a simulated surgery as part of their examination during which their performance in dealing with the problems presented would be observed and marked
- an objective structured clinical examination. This would consist of a series of tables or 'stations'. Candidates would spend time at each station and again be observed and marked. The stations might be task orientated (e.g. involving taking blood pressure or examining fundi), may look at consultation skills with an actor playing the part of a patient, or could be organisational (e.g. what are the mistakes on this patient's sick certificate?).

The debate is now not whether there should be a clinical component but what form it should take. Whatever the form, the component will have to test what the examiners feel are the priority areas not currently tested adequately elsewhere by the examination, be reliable and above all be practical given the numbers of candidates involved.

## Why do candidates fail the examination?

The first thing to say is that failing does not indicate that one is a 'bad' doctor or even an inadequate general practitioner. Failing indicates that one was not in the top 72–74% of the candidates sitting the examination – nothing more and nothing less. Most experienced general practitioners know of competent and caring colleagues who have failed the MRCGP. Doctors are not used to failing at many things, particularly examinations, and the MRCGP examination is likely to come in for criticism unfairly when this occurs. One would not say that 26–28% of British general practitioners (the percentage who fail the examination) should not be GPs and being in this peer group is no disgrace. The examination is not assessing who should or should not be general practitioners. It merely passes approximately the top three-quarters of those sitting the test. If one finds oneself in the bottom quarter it may be for one, some or all of the following reasons.

1. Missing the train, the car breaking down, sleeping in or some other reason for arriving late. Obvious but sadly still true. It happens most years to someone at either the written papers or the orals.

2. Failing to read the instructions on the paper. Also obvious but it still happens.

3. Answering a different question from that asked. The examiners will not be able to offer any marks in this situation. If the question asks about the evidence for the usefulness of *screening* for hypertension there are no marks for discussing the *management* of hypertension.

4. Inadequate preparation. This manifests itself either as unfamiliarity with the current literature of general practice (no reading) or with the content or aims of the examination. Candidates with acceptable approaches, knowledge bases and attitudes still fail the examination through not having their skills organised and practised in a way in which they can demonstrate them to the examiners.

5. An inadequate knowledge base. This is mainly measured in the MCQ paper. A really poor performance means that there is a lot of ground to be made up in the other two written papers. This is possible but difficult. Even then, further deficiencies are likely to be uncovered in the oral examination.

6. Lack of reading. This may be a problem in the MCQ paper since it results in a lack of factual knowledge. The CRQ paper is designed specifically to look at the breadth and depth of reading. In the vivas it is not possible for candidates to score more than a bare pass unless they can justify at least some of the stated management with reference to the published literature.

7. Too narrow or doctor-centred medicine. The examiners believe in discussing the patient's ideas, concerns and expectations as a routine part of the consultation. Operating in the style of 'Take this and you will be better' is unlikely to find favour. Management options need to be multiple. Offering one approach as the one and only is unrealistic and unhelpful to patients. Dogmatism and authoritarianism are rarely appropriate in the examination or in general practice.

8. A lack of critical thought about patient management. Plans and current practices must be looked at critically and justified, again preferably with reference to the literature.

9. Lack of depth of knowledge with reference to practice organisation.

10. Lack of thought when prescribing.

11. Lack of appropriate organisation and knowledge concerning the common chronic diseases.

12. Looking at problems only from the perspective of one's own experience. Handling a problem in the Yorkshire Dales may be a very different matter from handling the same problem in an inner city practice.

13. Failing to safely and appropriately handle emergency situations.

In 1985 the desirable and undesirable attributes of general practitioners were focused upon by the examiners. After much refining, the following groups of desirable characteristics were produced. These are the attributes the examination seeks to test. If candidates do not possess them or fail to demonstrate them to the examiners they may expect the consequences. Although the examiners were working originally with the oral examination in mind, the lists produced are applicable to the examination as a whole. From the candidate's point of view, this is what you will be tested on:

### A. CLINICAL COMPETENCE

1. Ability to diagnose and manage life-threatening problems in general practice.
2. Possession of an adequate knowledge base and the ability to apply it.
3. Problem solving abilities:
   a. Recognising and understanding the whole of the patient's presenting problem.
   b. Applying probabilities logically, selecting what is urgent and important.
   c. Considering options and alternatives.
   d. Thoughtful prescribing and an awareness of the dangers of medical intervention.
4. Care of the whole patient and the family, including psychological and social dimensions.
5. Rational planning for the management of chronic disease.
6. Ability to diagnose and manage common psychological problems in general practice.
7. Interest in and ability to achieve effective preventative medicine.

### B. PRACTICE ORGANISATION

1. Willingness and ability to be accessible in his/her practice.
2. Interest in teamwork and appreciation of the role of other health workers.
3. Ability to generate priorities in practice management.
4. Ability to use time effectively and appropriately.
5. Ability to use resources appropriately.

### C. COMMUNICATION

1. Understanding the importance of communicating between patients and doctors.
2. Ability to communicate effectively.

3. Willingness and ability to seek patients' health beliefs.
4. Acceptance of the role of the general practitioner as an educator.

### D. PROFESSIONAL VALUES

1. Respect for human life.
2. Empathy and a willingness to care.
3. Sensitivity and awareness of patients' attitudes and problems.
4. Respect for patients as people, not disease processes.
5. Flexibility and a respect for others, including cultural tolerance.
6. Willingness to take responsibility for personal and continuing care of patients.
7. Reliability and conscientiousness.
8. Integrity and an appreciation of the ethical and moral aspects of practice, including confidentiality.
9. Enjoyment and enthusiasm in his/her work.

### E. PERSONAL AND PROFESSIONAL GROWTH

1. Awareness of his or her own attitudes and feelings and the effect of these.
2. Willingness to examine his/her own work and limitations.
3. Ability to think clearly and critically and to justify decisions.
4. Awareness of the difficulties in balancing personal and professional life.
5. Involvement in continuing education.

Being even more helpful, the examiners have actually published their list of those attributes that they felt were worthy of particular attention in future examinations:

1. Safety in dealing with emergency situations.

2. Understanding communications between doctors and patients.

5

3. Ability to plan the management of chronic diseases.
4. Interest in teamwork.
5. Practice of continuity of care.
6. Accessibility.
7. Fulfilment of commitments.
8. Ability to evaluate own work critically.
9. Awareness of limitations.
10. Interest in standards of care.
11. Seeking of health beliefs of patients.
12. Evidence of critical reading and familiarity with literature.
13. Evidence of continuing education.

Candidates planning their study programmes might profit from using these lists as a skeleton to organise reading and revision.

Many candidates benefit from attending an MRCGP preparation course. Some examiners are concerned that this may result in candidates being excessively coached but the majority attitude may be deduced from the fact that the RCGP collates details of courses and will on request furnish candidates with a list. From experience, most potential candidates who have attended our Yorkshire course depart very doubtful about their chances of performing to their maximum potential without the course and are very glad to have taken part. Those who have attended a variety of courses say that those lasting 2 or 3 days and involving group work offer greater benefit than those of shorter duration. As a peer group referenced examination it is essential to know where one stands in one's peer group as revision commences.

The timing of revision and attending a preparation course requires some planning. A minimum of 8–10 weeks steady academic work is required by the majority of candidates prior to the examination. A preparation course 2 weeks before sitting the written papers may provide some insight into technique but no real chance to practise, and for most will be a waste of time, effort and money. The MRCGP examination is a serious professional examination and deserves respect. It is, however, eminently passable by most candidates and more still would pass if preparation was better organised.

# 2
# Revision Programme

With such a vast range of literature to consult and limited time available each candidate will have to decide their priorities. The first task is to find out what the MRCGP examination is setting out to test and why. Detailed descriptions of the examination's development are contained in the section 'Aims and Objectives' and in Occasional Paper 46 published by the RCGP.

Sensible progress can then be made by moving on to see how much revision needs to be done and in what areas by looking at past papers. These are available from the RCGP and there are also several excellent books of practice papers published which have the advantage of model answers. There are also opportunities in this workbook to try practice papers.

The hard work of reading, revising and practising examination techniques can then begin. The following is an example of the study programme a conscientious candidate might construct. It is intended only as an example of a type of structured approach and should not be followed slavishly since each of us is an individual with our own individual educational needs.

## Time available

Assume 12 weeks study time prior to written examinations and 6 weeks between written papers and orals.

Before written papers:
- *Weekdays* Assume 1 night on call, 1 night recovering/relaxing/socialising.
  Plan, therefore, 4 hours × 3 nights × 12 weeks.
- *Weekends* Assume 2 weekends on call, 2 weekends off. During revision weekends plan for 8 hours study each day, still leaving time for family, friends, shopping, laundry etc.
  Plan, therefore, for 8 weekends, 8 hours per day.
- *Total* 144 hours during the week, 128 hours at weekends.

Candidates are often surprised at the amount of time available once some structure is imposed and if the timetable can be adhered to. With 248 hours before the written examinations the volume of reading begins to look manageable.

After written papers:
- *Weekdays* Plan for 4 hours $\times$ 3 nights/week $\times$ 6 weeks.
- *Weekends* Plan for 4 hours per day $\times$ 4 weekends.
- *Total* 104 hours

If all MRCGP candidates were to put in 476 hours of appropriate revision the examiners might have to pass more than the present 72–74%. Candidates should note that this timetable leaves plenty of time for activities other than work and the MRCGP examination.

## Resources

It is surprising how often medical graduates, who have by definition passed many examinations, fail to pay significant attention to basic educational needs. A quiet comfortable place to study is an obvious priority. Access to refreshments and yet avoidance of easy distractions should be considered. Friends, family and all colleagues need to be consulted and informed of the study plan as a matter of courtesy. However attractive it may seem to prepare and sit the examination whilst keeping friends and colleagues unaware in case of failure, the chances of success, which are already quite good, will be vastly increased with a large support group all prepared to help, swap duties and generally be considerate for the 12 weeks of intensive study.

Books, papers and journals can be acquired from a variety of sources. Candidates have sometimes had difficulty obtaining some references. Try the libraries of the training practices in your area or the local postgraduate medical library if you have one. The British Medical Association (BMA) and RCGP libraries offer a superb service to their members and associate members respectively. Becoming an associate member of the RCGP may not only provide access to library facilities but could save the successful candidate money for the first year after passing the examination. Successful candidates who are already associate members of the College do not need to pay their first year's College membership fees. The British Library at Boston Spa should be able to track down absolutely everything if all fails. They will even locate references and reserve you a reading room to work in if you communicate with them and give reasonable notice.

Often it is the government leaflets and publications that are the hardest to locate. HMSO Publications Centre can be contacted at PO Box 276, London SW8 5DT or HMSO Books, Dept B, FREEPOST, Norwich NR3 1BR. The London Centre accepts telephone orders with Visa, Mastercard and American Express, Tel. 071-873 9090. Alternatively fax orders to 071-873 8200.

Locating references, obtaining photocopies of articles, and tracking down books and pamphlets can be very time consuming. Candidates should be reading the material not finding it. The latter task should be delegated, and the most likely victims are the post-graduate centre librarian or the practice secretary. It is vital to give them time to obtain the documents you require. There are only a finite number of copies available of any given text and orders may take time to arrive. Popular titles may be in the hands of others as the examinations approach and it may be worthwhile obtaining all of one's requirements early in the revision period. Some may not be obtainable on loan and if the cost is moderate and the source a key one, then a small personal investment in its purchase may be well worthwhile. Ask politely for assistance from whoever can do your searching for you, give them accurate titles and references to look for and reward them with a small gift when the pass is obtained.

## Revision curriculum

### 1. Examination content and technique

- Palmer K T 1992 Notes for the MRCGP, 2nd edn. Blackwell Scientific Publications, Oxford

- Examination for membership of the Royal College of General Practitioners 1990 Development, current state and future needs. RCGP Occasional Paper 46

- Murray T S 1986 Modified essay questions for the MRCGP. Blackwell Scientific Publications, Oxford

- Gambrill E, Moulds A, Fry J, Brooks D 1988 The MRCGP study book, 2nd edn. Butterworths/Update

  Oxford GP Group 1987 A guide to general practice, 2nd edn. Blackwell Scientific Publications, Oxford

- Green, Sanderson and Ferguson 1991 MCQs for the MRCGP. Kluwer

- McGuinnes B 1987 MCQs in general practice, 2nd edn. Mark Allen Publishers. Available only from Publishers: 081-671 7521

- Elliott P G 1989 MRCGP – MCQs. Springer-Verlag

Keith Palmer has written a wonderful book which is, in most people's opinion, the single most useful resource when preparing for the MRCGP. The second edition is mandatory, however, since some sections in the first edition are now out of date.

## 2. Clinical medicine

It takes a minimum of 3 years of full-time study to cover the undergraduate clinical curriculum. Obviously it is unrealistic and unnecessary for most candidates to even consider revision over a wide range of the clinical spectrum. Areas of weakness need identifying and concentration on the special problems that only present to general practitioners is usually rewarding. The following books will refresh the mind, broaden approaches and reinforce attitudes towards good general practice and for many are a useful starting point:

- Cormack J, Marinker M, Morrell D 1987 Practice – a handbook of primary medical care. Churchill Livingstone, Edinburgh

- Sandars J E, Baron R 1988 Learning general practice – a structured approach for trainee GPs and trainers. PasTest Service

Particular attention should be paid to management of chronic diseases in general practice, management of common general practice problems (e.g. sore throats, diarrhoea and vomiting) and rational, thoughtful prescribing policies with alternative options available. As you read, work all the time on formulating personal management plans, putting each nugget of information into place in an appropriate priority rating bearing in mind options, implications and choice.

For those candidates involved in vocational training, identification of areas of weakness may already be part of an ongoing assessment of progress as part of the region's VTS programme.

Even if they have this advantage most candidates could learn from doing a number of mock examinations under realistic conditions. A consistent pattern of poor scores in some areas of these may show where extra concentration is needed and revision of a recent edition of a short textbook in those specialities may be required.

e.g. Lecture Notes in ........ (Blackwell)

    ABC of .......... (BMJ)

The *Medicine International* series is excellent as a source of facts for improving the database if the MCQ is proving a particular problem in clinical areas.

Therapeutics revision should be adequately covered by reading or re-reading the latest edition of the British National Formulary.

Some candidates have initial poor MEQ scores because of too narrow an approach. Think all the time when revising not of what you **would** do but of what you **might** do. This may be practised and reinforced perhaps most usefully in discussions with other doctors – either through a local MRCGP study group or through informal regular discussions of problem cases in the practice which can open up the candidate who tends to be too doctor-centred.

### 3. Critical reading

The examination guidelines recommend the following as adequate preparation:

- Gore S M, Altman D G 1982 Statistics in practice. BMA, pp 1–24

- 1990 Guidelines for writing papers. BMJ 300: 38–40

- Jewell D 1988 Reading scientific articles or how to cope with the overload. Practitioner 232: 720–725

- Sackett D L, Hayes R B, Tugwell P 1985 Clinical epidemiology: a basic science for clinical medicine. Little, Brown and Co., Boston and Toronto

- Swinscow T D V 1981 Statistics at square one, 3rd edn. BMA

However, many people find that 'Simple Statistics' by Frances Clegg, published by the Cambridge University Press, is the first book on statistics that makes any sense. Frances Clegg is a psychologist and therefore writes in terms that those of us in the biological sciences are familiar with, whereas other books with the same aim are written by mathematicians who often relapse into their own language which is about as intelligible as Latin to most modern medical postgraduates.

Journals need to be read to develop a personal database to cover Question 2 in the critical reading paper. The following ought to provide an adequate selection:

BMJ } These are mandatory for the CRQ.

BJGP } The last 2 years' issues MUST be read.

Update

Drug and Therapeutics Bulletin

Medeconomics

Pulse/General Practitioner/Doctor

Practitioner

When reading the journals it pays to create a 'keyword index'. A single word or a short phrase, usually from the title, is used to create an index card. Examples might be diabetes, consultation length/behaviour, new contract. As the reading progresses each index card will expand to include other references to papers on the same subject. Further revision can then be directed to re-reading of groups of papers on the same subject to gain an overall state-of-the-art picture of current knowledge and opinion in that area. A similar system has been used to create the grouped references to papers in this book and they may serve as examples.

### 4. Other reading

Reading the journals can be broken up with other material that can be conveniently divided into three groups:

#### a. Classic textbooks of British general practice

- BMA & Pharmaceutical Society of Great Britain. British National Formulary

- Fry J/RCGP 1979 Trends in general practice, 2nd edn. RCGP

- Fry J/RCGP 1983 Present state and future needs, 6th edn. MTP Press

- Hodgkin K 1985 Towards earlier diagnosis, 5th edn. Churchill Livingstone, Edinburgh

- DHSS/Byrne, Long 1976 Doctors talking to patients. HMSO

- Balint M 1968 The doctor, his patient and the illness, 2nd edn. Pitman

- Pendleton et al. 1984 The consultation. Oxford General Practice Series.

- Neighbour R The inner consultation. Kluwer Academic Publishers

- Berne E 1968 Games people play. Penguin

- Fry J 1985 Common diseases, their nature, incidence and care, 4th edn. MTP Press

- Moulds, Martin, Bouchier-Hayes 1985 Emergencies in general practice, 2nd edn. MTP Press

- Tudor Hart J 1988 A new kind of doctor. Merlin Press Ltd

### b. Government publications

DoH/DHSS

- Joint Committee on Vaccination 1992
  Immunisation against infectious disease
  HMSO

- Summary of the Mental Health Act 1983,
  Reprinted 1986

- Medical evidence for statutory sick,
  pay, statutory maternity pay and social
  security incapacity benefit purposes
  Revised 1991

- Medical aspects of fitness to drive,
  4th edn. 1985

- Handbook of contraceptive practice,
  1990 edn.

- Guide to the Misuse of Drugs Act
  1985 No: 2066

- The quality of medical care, 1990 HMSO

- Drug misuse and dependence, 1991 DoH,
  Scottish & Welsh Guidelines on clinical
  management, HMSO

Office of Health Economics

- George Teeling Smith 1991
  Patterns of prescribing

### c. RCGP publications

The RCGP produces a series of reports, occasional papers and information folders. The prudent candidate should study these closely – a list of current publications is obtainable directly from Princes Gate.

This looks initially a formidable list but none of the government and RCGP publications are very lengthy. It should be possible to get through several of these in an evening's work. Enthusiastic candidates working steadily can easily read and make revision notes on three or four of the shorter classic textbooks of general practice in a single week using the above revision schedule.

## 5. Between the written and oral examinations

Candidates must assume that they have performed well enough on the written papers to be called for the vivas. There is never enough time to do everything as the written papers approach and few candidates will suffer in the written papers by leaving some of the classic textbooks of general practice unread until this period.

There is much to be gained by viva practice (see 'The Orals'), further reading of the journals and polishing of references. As the orals approach keep up to date particularly with the current journals. All of the examiners are GPs under pressure and will be catching up with their reading at the last minute. It is likely, therefore, that they will have picked up the latest batch of journals from the hall table and hope to impress both candidates and fellow examiners with how up to date they are with their reading – most of it having been done on the train on the way to the examination! Even examiners cram.

# 3
# The Multiple Choice Question Paper

- Format
- Content
- Technique
- MCQ Paper I
  — Questions
  — Answers
- MCQ Paper II
  — Questions
  — Answers

## Format

Most candidates are experienced in multiple choice question examinations. For many the MCQ paper is the most disliked of the three written papers but in fact the marks scored by candidates are often better than anticipated.

Two hours are allocated for 360 questions. Each question has a short main stem and is followed by a variable number of branches. Candidates are required to decide whether each branch is true or false. In most British MCQ papers, it is possible for candidates to leave blank branches, or indeed whole questions which they are unable to answer. Negative marking USUALLY operates with $+1$ for a correct answer, $-1$ for an incorrect answer and 0 if no answer is provided.

However, **from the autumn papers of 1992 the MRCGP examiners abandoned negative marking**. The scoring is now, therefore, $+1$ for a correct answer, 0 for a blank or incorrect answer. Some revision of examination technique will therefore be required by most candidates.

A number of MCQ questions in variable formats have also been introduced. Read the instructions carefully.

## Content

Until 1992 the distribution of questions between specialities was as follows:

| | |
|---|---|
| General medicine | 10 |
| Therapeutics | 6 |
| Surgical diagnosis | 3 |
| Traumatology | 2 |
| Infectious diseases | 2 |
| Care of the elderly | 2 |
| Paediatrics | 5 |
| Psychiatry | 6 |
| Obstetrics/gynaecology | 6 |
| Dermatology | 4 |
| Ophthalmology | 4 |
| ENT | 2 |
| Legal/ethical | 2 |
| Epidemiology/research methods | 2 |
| Practice organisation | 4 |

The examiners now have reserved the right to modify this distribution, although radical changes would seem to be unlikely, at least initially. The content has been refined over the years and occasionally modifications have been introduced to raise the profile of an area within the curriculum of general practice. The introduction of medico-legal questions is a good example of this policy.

Until 1992 the MCQ paper was set out in the above specialty order i.e. questions 1–10 were always general medicine, questions 11–16 were therapeutics and so on. This is not now the case and subject matter will be random throughout the paper.

The College uses specific terms and definitions when setting multiple choice questions. It is vital for candidates to study the following and practise MCQs which use these phrases in order to be using the same language as the examiners when sitting down to the paper.

| | |
|---|---|
| **Characteristic** | Implies a feature of such diagnostic significance that its absence would cast doubt on the diagnosis. |
| **Typical** | Implies a feature that one would expect to be present but perhaps not so diagnostically absolute as 'characteristic'. |
| **Recognised** | Implies a fact that has been reliably reported and which a candidate would be expected to know without the fact being either characteristic or typical. |
| **Has been shown** | Implies information which has been repeated so often as to gain an accolade of accepted truth or can be demonstrated by reference to an authoritative paper on the subject. |

By judicious use of questions originating with short stems and sticking rigidly to these definitions, the examiners usually manage to produce a question paper with fewer ambiguities than the usual MCQ paper. There is a bank of questions but 30% of the questions are new on each occasion. An item correctly answered by 95% of candidates in an examination is unlikely to be used again.

The general standard set is taxing but not unreasonable. Some candidates, particularly mature candidates perhaps, become lulled into a comfortable mental armchair when consulted by scores of grateful patients each week who regard them as an expert on matters as widely divergent as the pros and cons of coronary artery by-pass grafting and the correct age for a daughter to begin wearing a bra! Before commencing practice MCQ examinations it is important to realise that hardly any general practitioner is good enough to achieve more than about 80% in the MCQ paper. Many excellent general practitioners do well to achieve crude scores of 70% so do not despair if initial scores are a blow to the ego.

## Technique

1. Candidates are presented with a question paper, an answer sheet, a 2B pencil and a rubber. Write your name and candidates number clearly on the answer sheet.

2. Like many large multiple choice papers, the marking is greatly simplified by the use of technology. The answer paper is passed through a photoelectric cell which reads each small answer 'lozenge'. If you think an answer to be true carefully shade in that lozenge. If it is false, then shade in the false lozenge.

3. Use the 2B pencil provided to do the shading. Another grade of pencil, felt tip or ink will give the marking system problems.

4. If you change your mind about an answer, be sure to use the rubber provided to erase the original shading completely or again, problems will result.

5. Read each stem in conjunction with each branch individually and come to a decision as to your answer about that question individually.

6. There is plenty of time for most candidates in the MCQ paper. Read the stem and branch carefully and with reference to the definitions provided above. Many marks have been lost by answering a similar question rather than the actual one that the examiners have set. For example, don't confuse endometritis with endometriosis.

7. From experience, it is usually wise to answer provisionally in rough on the question paper. As you reach the end of each set of branches transfer your answer to the lozenges en bloc and then turn to the next question, answer in rough, transfer and so on. This method minimises the risk of filling in the wrong lozenge. Time is rarely a problem in the MCQ paper but it would be a disaster to have carefully sketched out a set of immaculate answers in rough only to run out of time before transferring the pearls of knowledge to the answer sheet and gaining the due marks. The additional advantage of transferring one question at a time is the ability to monitor your rate of progress through the paper.

There are very few candidates who can work their way through a MCQ paper, provide an answer to 75% of the questions on the basis that they are sure that each answer is correct and walk out of the examination hall with an air of supreme confidence.

Most of us are ordinary mortals. The examination now recognises this and with the abolition of negative marking the MCQ paper rewards achievement and the possession of knowledge rather than punishing ignorance.

It is therefore mandatory to answer all the questions on the MCQ paper. This will require what many would view as blind guessing. However, on MRCGP courses I have been involved with we have regularly had candidates improve their performance in negatively marked MCQs by more than 20% when they were forced to answer all questions! What we are dealing with is not random guessing. This is (quite seriously) intelligent guessing which is a combination of subconscious and conscious recall with a bit of professional intuition, and sometimes involves working through to an answer from almost forgotten basic sciences.

Do not, therefore, be afraid to dig deeply when faced with a question that at first sight you have little idea about. Somewhere you may just have a little inkling, perhaps almost a hunch – often one's first thought is the best in those circumstances.

Some practice is required at this technique. The RCGP does not release past MCQ papers but there are a number of books containing appropriate practice examinations. Individual candidates would be well advised to go through some of the papers and see whether they score best and are most comfortable answering questions in strict order. The alternative is to quickly answer those branches they are very confident about first and then think long and hard about the less obvious sections. This is a very individual matter and may make a small but significant difference in marks gained. Only trying each method out will reveal which is best for you.

Do remember each time you come across 'characteristic', 'recognised', 'typical' and 'has been shown' that these phrases have very specific meanings in the MRCGP MCQ paper. Examples of this influence follow in the two practice papers. Candidates wishing to compare their performance with their peers might be interested to know that performance in recent preparation courses using these papers resulted in a mean of 73%. The abolition of negative marking has resulted in a very small standard deviation of 7% and therefore candidates scoring less than 66% on these papers would need to prepare particularly conscientiously for this paper. It is *possible* to score somewhat below par on the MCQ paper and pick up enough marks on the other two written papers in order to be invited to the oral part of the examination. However, without wishing to make too sweeping a generalisation, it is rare to find a candidate well below one standard deviation from the mean on the MCQ paper and well above the mean on the other papers. It would seem that an adequate knowledge base is mostly constructed from regular reading and this has benefits in the other papers.

Finally, a word of encouragement. The MCQ paper is only 33% of the available marks in the written papers and only 20% of the total marks in the MRCGP examination as a whole. Some candidates may become disillusioned when sitting the written papers if they find the MCQ, as the first paper, very difficult. Remember that a number of questions and branches in the MCQ paper are designed very much to sort out the really exceptional candidate from the rest of us. Do not, therefore, get flustered. Use the interval between papers to keep cool, calm and dispassionate in the face of apparent disaster in order to produce your best performance in the other two written papers to follow.

# Multiple Choice Question Paper I

## Instructions to candidates:
1. There are 100 questions on this paper.
2. Time allowed: 30 minutes.
3. Indicate your answer on the question paper i.e.True/False.
4. Answer all questions.

**Absolute contraindictions to the combined oral contraceptive include:**
1. Porphyria
2. Dubin Johnson syndrome
3. Lactation.
4. Hypertension.
5. Secondary amenorrhoea.

**The following drugs are benzodiazepines considered to be short acting in comparison to intermediate and long acting:**
6. Nitrazepam.
7. Lorazepam.
8. Clobazam.
9. Temazepam.
10. Triazolam.

**The following statements regarding FP10 prescriptions and controlled drugs are correct:**
11. A prescription is valid for 6 months from the date thereon.
12. All doctors may prescribe Schedule I drugs as defined in the Misuse of Drugs Regulations 1985.
13. It is not a criminal offence for a doctor to issue an incomplete prescription.
14. A prescription for phenobarbitone must be written in the doctor's handwriting.
15. Under no circumstances can a general practitioner prescribe diamorphine to a diamorphine addict.

**In Paget's disease of bone:**
16. There are areas of bone with dense and disorganised sclerosis.
17. High output cardiac failure is a recognised complication.
18. Areas of Paget's are more likely to be the site of metastases than normal bone.
19. The serum alkaline phosphatase is characteristically elevated.
20. Serum calcium is typically elevated.

**In Parkinson's disease:**
21. The primary cause may be syphilitic mesencephalitis.
22. Subnormal weight is a characteristic feature.
23. Anticholinergic drugs are effective against bradykinesia.
24. Hallucinations are a recognised side effect of levo-dopa therapy.
25. Idiopathic Parkinson's disease shortens life expectancy.

**In non-insulin dependent diabetics:**
26. Polygenic inheritance is characteristic.
27. Hyperinsulinaemia may occur.
28. Glycosylated haemoglobin reflects the level of blood glucose over the previous 4 weeks.
29. Sulphonylurea hypoglycaemic coma is more likely if the patient is also taking $\beta$-blocking drugs.
30. Diabetic nephropathy is typically accompanied by proliferative retinopathy.

**When assuming a diagnosis of benign breast disease the GP should be aware that:**
31. Cysts are found typically after the menopause.
32. Distortion of the breast is characteristic of fibroadenosis.
33. Gynaecomastia in adult males is a recognised feature of untreated prostatic carcinoma.

34. Cyclical mastitis typically affects the medial half of the breast.
35. Discharge from multiple orifices on the nipple is characteristic of intraduct carcinoma.

**The following findings are typical of a baby at birth born normally at 40 weeks gestation:**
36. Absent walking reflex.
37. Lies prone with knees drawn up under abdomen.
38. Incomplete head lag when pulled to sitting position.
39. On ventral suspension head maintained in same horizontal plane as rest of body.
40. Hands clenched.

**In simple febrile convulsions:**
41. The child is aged 6 months to 7 years.
42. Fever is always present.
43. The fit may be generalised or focal.
44. Recurrence risk is greater if the first fit is before 18 months of age.
45. Temporal lobe epilepsy is a recognised secondary effect.

**Absolute contraindications to pertussis vaccination are:**
46. Cerebral palsy.
47. Spina bifida.
48. A fever of 40°C within 48 hours of a previous pertussis immunisation.
49. Snuffles.
50. Neonatal jaundice.

**The following features are characteristic of puerperal psychosis:**
51. Onset within 10 days of delivery.
52. Previous history of psychiatric illness.
53. Family history of psychiatric illness.
54. Affective disorder.
55. Recurrence following future pregnancies.

**In anorexia nervosa:**
56. Developing social isolation is an early feature.
57. Disturbance of body image is characteristic.
58. Amenorrhoea occurs typically early in the developing syndrome.
59. There is an association with impulsive behaviour such as shoplifting.

60. The long term prognosis is characteristically good.

**In secondary amenorrhoea:**
61. Due to hyperprolactinaemia, galactorrhoea is a characteristic feature.
62. Imperforate hymen is a recognised cause.
63. Following cessation of oral contraceptive therapy, spontaneous resumption of menstruation within 12 months is characteristic.
64. Elevated serum FSH suggests ovarian failure.
65. Appropriately treated by clomiphene, menstruation characteristically occurs within 8 days of stopping the clomiphene.

**Absolute and relative contraindications to insertion of an IUCD include:**
66. Anticoagulant therapy.
67. Long-term treatment with steroids.
68. Cervical erosion.
69. Previous ectopic pregnancy.
70. Active monilial vaginosis.

**The following occur in psoriasis:**
71. Onycholysis.
72. Scaling lesions.
73. Koebner phenomenon.
74. Rapid relapse after stopping topical steroids.
75. Sparing of palms and soles.

**Anterior uveitis:**
76. Is a recognised cause of glaucoma.
77. Typically presents with circumcorneal vasodilatation.
78. Associated with Still's disease typically gives hyphaema.
79. Is a recognised association of ankylosing spondylitis.
80. Responds rapidly to topical antibiotics.

**Otalgia is a recognised feature of:**
81. A C4-5 disc lesion.
82. Osteoarthrosis of the temporo-mandibular joint.
83. Tonsillitis.
84. Carcinoma of posterior third of tongue.
85. Chronic suppurative otitis media.

**When evaluating clinical trials:**

86. A very small probability value suggests that the null hypothesis should be rejected.
87. A wide confidence interval reflects an inadequate sample size.
88. A Chi squared test cannot be used to estimate the required sample size.
89. Regression to the mean should be remedied by repeated 'run in' observations.
90. Comparisons generated by the data, rather than specified in advance, increase the credibility of the trial.

**Under his terms of service a GP who is offering unrestricted services shall:**

91. Offer a consultation at the surgery to any patient I6–74 years of age who has not attended any consultation within the previous 3 years.
92. Offer an annual domiciliary visit to each patient aged 75 years and above.
93. Arrange compulsory in-service training for ancillary staff.
94. Live within a radius of 10 miles of the main practice premises.
95. Provide general medical services spread over 4 days/week if the 5th day is spent practising industrial medicine.

**According to the statement of fees and allowances:**

96. A fee is payable for children under 15 years of age for child health surveillance (CHS) services provided the GP is on the CHS register.
97. A GP may claim a temporary resident fee and a night visit fee if called to see a temporary resident at 22.30 hours.
98. For calculation of immunisation for children aged 2 years and under, diphtheria and polio are considered to be in the same group.
99. For cervical cytology purposes a GP would have reached the upper target when he has smeared 70% of the women in his practice between the ages of 25 and 64 within the last 5.5 years.
100. A GP can claim a fee for administering cholera vaccine to a woman who is travelling to an infected area.

# MCQ Answers
## Paper I

1. True    – Handbook of Contraceptive Practice 1990 p 28
2. True
3. False
4. False
5. False
6. False    – Monthly Index Medical Specialties Jan 91 p 77.
7. False
8. False
9. False
10. True
11. False    – BNF: Guidance on Prescribing Controlled Drugs
12. False
13. False
14. False
15. False
16. True    – Oxford textbook of medicine (OTM) 17.19
17. True
18. True
19. True
20. False
21. True    – OTM–21.221
22. True
23. False
24. True
25. True
26. True    – OTM–9.51
27. True
28. False
29. True
30. True
31. False    – Reid D.J. Update 1988 36(7) 2046
32. False
33. False
34. False
35. False
36. False    – Illingworth : Basic Developmental Screening 0–4 years
37. True
38. False
39. False
40. True
41. False    – Community Paediatrics Polnay/ Hull Chapter 11
42. True
43. False
44. True
45. True
46. False    – Immunisation Against Infectious Disease 1992 I IMSO
47. False
48. True
49. False
50. False
51. True    – Medicine International 1987 (44) 1814
52. False
53. False
54. True
55. False
56. True    – Medicine International 1987(45) 1846
57. True
58. False
59. True
60. False
61. False    – Medicine International 1984 (12) 513
62. False
63. True
64. True

**65.** False

**66.** True      – Handbook of Contraceptive
                      Practice 1990 HMSO

**67.** True
**68.** False
**69.** True
**70.** True

**71.** True      – Medicine International 1988 (49)
                      2012

**72.** True
**73.** True
**74.** True
**75.** False

**76.** True      – OTM-23.8
**77.** True
**78.** False
**79.** True
**80.** False

**81.** False     – ABC of ENT Chapter 1
**82.** True
**83.** True
**84.** True
**85.** False

**86.** True      – Medicine International 1988 (59)
                      2451

**87.** True
**88.** False
**89.** True
**90.** False

**91.** True      – Terms of Service for Doctors in
                      General Practice Nov 1989

**92.** True
**93.** False
**94.** False
**95.** False

**96.** False    – Statement of Fees and Allow-
                      ances 1990

**97.** True
**98.** True
**99.** False
**100.** True

# Multiple Choice Question Paper II

## Instructions to candidates:
1. There are 100 questions on this paper.
2. Time allowed: 30 minutes.
3. Indicate your answer on the question paper i.e.True/False.
4. Answer all questions.

**The following are recognised features of lithium toxicity:**
1. Cerebellar dysfunction.
2. Muscle twitching.
3. Decreased level of consciousness.
4. Cardiac arrhythmias.
5. Constipation.

**The following pairs of drugs interact with clinical significance:**
6. Alcohol and Metronidazole.
7. Dothiepin and Terfenadine.
8. Metformin and Atenolol.
9. Frusemide and Fenbufen.
10. Digoxin and Erythromycin.

**Appropriate advice on fitness to drive a private motor vehicle would include:**
11. Do not drive within 2 months after recovery from a myocardial infarct.
12. A long history of angina provoked only by avoidable effort is not sufficient reason to stop driving.
13. Controlled atrial fibrillation in the absence of heart disease is not a driving hazard.
14. One-eyed drivers must inform the DVLC of their disability.
15. Patients suffering from psychotic illness should inform the DVLC if the condition is likely to last more than 3 months.

**In ulcerative colitis:**
16. Age of onset is typically after puberty.
17. Anal fistula development is more likely than in Crohn's disease.
18. Most patients are non-smokers.
19. The risk of carcinomatous change is greater when the colon is very extensively involved.
20. Diagnosis may be confused with Chlamydia proctitis.

**It is true to say of coronary artery disease that:**
21. An ECG after myocardial infarct and discharge from hospital is a good prognostic indicator.
22. An inferior infarct diagnosed by ECG has a more favourable prognosis than anterior infarction.
23. The prognosis is better in asymptomatic patients than in symptomatic patients.
24. Half of deaths from myocardial infarction occur within 2 hours of onset of symptoms.
25. The risk of death after infarction is increased by the presence of bradycardia.

**Ectopic cardiac rhythm is a recognised feature of:**
26. Viral illness.
27. Pregnancy.
28. Excessive coffee intake.
29. Non-rheumatic heart valve disease.
30. Thyrotoxicosis.

**In congenital hypertrophic pyloric stenosis:**
31. Typically vomiting begins within 2 weeks of birth.
32. Chronic blood loss is a recognised complication.
33. Thickening the feed is one effective treatment.
34. Prognosis is better if operation is performed before rehydration.
35. When untreated, hypochloraemic alkalosis is a characteristic sequel.

23

**In the elderly, the following factors may increase the risk of pressure sores:**

36. Incontinence of urine.
37. Cerebrovascular accident.
38. Anaemia.
39. Hypoxia.
40. Peripheral vascular disease.

**Anterior dislocation of the shoulder:**

41. Is less common than posterior dislocation.
42. Is characteristically caused by a fall on the outstretched arm.
43. Causes considerable pain which is typically relieved by abducting the shoulder past about l00 degrees.
44. May be reduced using Hippocrates method.
45. May be complicated by injury to the accessory nerve.

**The following features indicate a good prognosis in schizophrenia:**

46. No obvious precipitating cause.
47. No family history of schizophrenia.
48. Gradual onset.
49. Stable work record.
50. Flattening of affect.

**Factors associated with an increased suicide risk after deliberate self-injury or self-poisoning include:**

51. Aged over 45 years.
52. Female sex.
53. Alcoholism.
54. Previous attempt involved a physical method e.g. drowning, hanging.
55. Criminal record

**The following maternal infections are recognised to cross the placenta:**

56. Varicella.
57. Treponema pallidum.
58. Cytomegalovirus.
59. Plasmodia.
60. Toxoplasma gondii.

**Factors suggesting that an antepartum haemorrhage at 34 weeks gestation was caused by placenta praevia include:**

61. Tender uterus.
62. Painless bleeding.
63. Transverse lie.
64. Previous bleeding in second trimester.
65. Maternal shock.

**Acne vulgaris is:**

66. Unknown in infancy.
67. Dependent on the level of circulating oestrogen.
68. A recognised cause of depigmentation in pigmented skin.
69. A recognised sequel to excessive use of cosmetics.
70. Effectively managed (if mild) by dietary restriction alone.

**Alopecia may be caused by:**

71. Trichotillomania.
72. Discoid lupus erythematosus.
73. Surgical shock.
74. Hypothyroidism.
75. Iron deficiency.

**In the differential diagnosis of a red eye:**

76. Circumcorneal injection is a sign of significant eye disease.
77. A normal pupil is characteristic of keratitis.
78. Generalised conjunctival congestion is typical of chronic simple glaucoma.
79. Keratic precipitates are typical of iritis.
80. Constriction of the pupil is a typical finding in anterior uveitis.

**Hearing loss is typically conductive when found in:**

81. Chronic suppurative otitis media.
82. Weavers.
83. Acoustic neuroma.
84. Aspirin overdose.
85. Middle ear effusion.

**In statistical terms:**

86. Transformation makes data conform more closely to a normal distribution using reciprocation.
87. The mode is the observation lying in the middle, when the observations are listed in increasing order.
88. In a skewed distribution the mode typically equals the mean.
89. 95% of observations fall within two standard deviations of the mean whatever the distribution.

90. The negative predictive value is the percentage of negatives which are true negatives.

**According to Statement of Fees and Allowances:**

91. A full post-natal care fee may be claimed if a patient leaves hospital within 48 hours of delivery.

92. A fee for emergency treatment applies to a person who is on the last day of a 2 week holiday.

93. To claim the maximum minor surgical fee 15 operations must be performed each quarter.

94. To claim rural practice units at least 30% of a GP's patients should be resident in a Rural Practice payment area.

95. Eligible practitioners under the Rent and Rates Scheme would be reimbursed 70% of their rent and 70% of their rates.

**Employment law necessitates:**

96. That employees receive a contract after 13 weeks of working for at least 16 hours/week.

97. Paid time off work for approved trade union duties.

98. Payment of redundancy pay after 52 weeks of continuous employment.

99. Notifications to Health and Safety executive if an employee fractures a femur whilst at work.

100. The offering of a pension scheme to full time employees.

# MCQ Answers
## Paper II

1. True    – Medicine International Jan 89 (61) 2530
2. True
3. True
4. True
5. False

6. True    – BNF. Appendix I.
7. True
8. True
9. True
10. True

11. True    – Medical Aspects of Fitness to Drive HMSO
12. True
13. True
14. True
15. True

16. True    – Medicine International Feb 86 (26) 1053
17. False
18. True
19. True
20. True

21. False    – Medicine International Aug 85 (20) 821
22. True
23. True

24. True
25. False

26. True    – Medicine International 1985 (17) 701
27. True
28. True
29. False
30. True

31. False    – OTM-12.140
32. False
33. False
34. False
35. True

36. True    – Coni, Davison, Webster. Lecture Notes on Geriatrics Ch. 9
37. True
38. True
39. True
40. True

41. False    – Apley AG. Apley's System of Orthopaedics and Fractures Ch 24
42. True
43. True
44. True
45. False

46. False    – Medicine International 1987 (43) 1773.
47. True
48. False
49. True
50. False

51. True    – Medicine International 1987 (43) 1786
52. False
53. True
54. True
55. False

56. True    – Kaye P. Notes for the DRCOG.
57. True
58. True
59. True
60. True

61. False    – Obstetrics by Ten Teachers. Clayton, Lewis & Pinker Ch.16
62. True
63. True
64. True

**65.** False

**66.** False – Medicine International 1988 (50) 2044

**67.** False
**68.** False
**69.** True
**70.** False

**71.** True – Medicine International 1988 (50) 2057

**72.** True
**73.** True
**74.** True
**75.** True

**76.** True – Essential ophthalmology. Hector, Bryson & Chawla Ch. 7

**77.** True
**78.** False
**79.** True
**80.** True

**81.** True – ABC of ENT p 10
**82.** False
**83.** False
**84.** False
**85.** True

**86.** False – Epidemiology in General Practice. Morrell D. p 41

**87.** False
**88.** False
**89.** False
**90.** True

**91.** True – Statement of Fees and Allowances 1990.

**92.** False
**93.** True
**94.** False
**95.** False

**96.** True – Palmer K. Notes for the MRCGP Ch.1

**97.** False
**98.** False
**99.** True
**100.** True

# 4

# The Modified Essay Question Paper

- Format
- Content
- Technique
- Practical points on technique
- MCQ practice paper
  — Questions
  — Answers

The Modified Essay Question (MEQ) paper was first developed by the MRCGP examiners. Its widespread adoption throughout vocational training as a teaching tool is a tribute to its success as an assessment technique, principally of the ability to take a broad approach to problems presented and to offer a range of potential options in treatment and help. Therefore, it is a test requiring some knowledge (clinical and organisational) and is quite an extensive test of attitudes.

## Format

The question paper consists of a booklet. Following the instructions to candidates there are a number of pages with the question posed at the top of each one. The rest of each page is left blank for the candidate's answer. Each page is stamped with the candidate's number and at the end of the examination the booklets are separated so that batches of pages can be dispatched to the examiners for marking. This has important consequences when considering the best strategy for answering the paper.

Two hours are allotted to answer the MEQ paper. The number of questions (pages) varies from one examination to the next and this is important when allocating time in the examination. The minimum number of pages is now 10, and two-part questions have fallen into disfavour. In years past the number of available marks could vary from page to page, which made the appropriate allocation of time even more difficult. Sensibly, the number of available marks per page is now the same.

## Content

In the past, succeeding question pages have either revealed an evolving story of a patient or family, or a number of unrelated problems which might form part of a GP's typical working day, or a combination of the two presentations. The vast majority of candidates now taking the examination are vocational trainees and the presentation of a series of family problems occurring over months or years will not, therefore, be within most candidates' experience.

The 'working day' approach also has the advantage of offering the examiners greater freedom in choosing the range of problems to present.

Candidates should be prepared for some novel material. In the recent past, for example, the examiners have asked candidates to write a referral letter, to comment on a patient's family tree and to discuss a protocol for a well-man clinic produced by their practice nurse. Ethical dilemmas and difficult or problem patients are popular.

The range of material commonly included is:

| | |
|---|---|
| **Clinical medicine** | Particularly chronic illness, prescribing and prevention. |
| **Problem patients** | Demanding or difficult personalities, unrealistic expectations, the effect of lifestyle on problem management, potential conflict, non-standard circumstances. |
| **Psychological problems** | Individual problems or family problems and the range of available treatment options. |
| **The consultation** | Particularly patient's ideas about their problems, their concerns and their own expectations. |
| **Practice organisation** | Particularly the Primary Health Care Team and practice administration. |
| **Relationship with colleagues** | Medical and paramedical. |
| **Hot or controversial topics** | There are always three or four topics currently under debate. |

## Practical points on technique

1. Write your name on the question paper and read the instructions to candidates carefully in case there has been a change you were not expecting.

2. Each page should have your candidate's number on it. Check that it has. If not, inform the invigilator.

3. Count the number of question sheets and divide your time between each question equally, allowing perhaps 10 minutes for leeway and reading through at the end. It is obvious with the use of a little simple arithmetic that a few additional marks gained from one or two extensively answered pages will be more than cancelled out if a candidate runs out of time and fails to attempt the last couple of pages.

4. Write legibly and in note form. Consider the plight of the average examiner. It is either the hottest weekend of the summer or a busy family time leading up to Christmas. The garden is in need of urgent resuscitation or there is a list of presents and cards that must be attended to. Suddenly, one evening you arrive home from an exhausting day and there it is – a large parcel from the RCGP containing 150 papers to be marked which you had forgotten all about! The only way to get through them is to make a large flask of coffee, wrap a wet towel around the forehead and make a start, often early in the morning or late at night. Contrary to popular opinion, the examiners are only human and in this entirely realistic scenario the legible, well set-out answer may attract that valuable few extra marks over the same answer written in an untidy scrawl that is difficult to read.

5. The question/answer booklet is separated out into separate pages after the examination so each examiner marks a pile of page 3s or a pile of page 7s, for example. You may, therefore, have to repeat information on separate pages and it is no use writing 'See page 5' because the examiner doing the marking can't! If there is an evolving story you may have to carry answers forwards or backwards. But a word of warning: only do so appropriately. For example, you may be asked for a list of differential diagnoses in a 15-year-old with headaches. Fair enough, but on the next page she turns out to have a glioma. It is not appropriate to backtrack and put glioma at the top of the list because space-occupying lesions are an incredibly rare cause of headaches presented to general practitioners.

6. Write 'PTO' very boldly if you fill the answer page and are turning over to write more on the back of that page.

7. Read the question posed very carefully and answer exactly the question which has been asked. If you are asked about the *problems* created for the *family* of a 34-year-old mother of two who is terminally ill with leukaemia there will only be marks for *family problems*. An exemplary thesis on the side effects of the patient's chemotherapy may contain a wealth of accurate information but may gain no marks at all. If it is relevant, write it down. If it isn't – don't!

8. It may be necessary to state the obvious. For example, if asked to describe the procedure for injecting a tennis elbow it is necessary to explain that one would ask the patient to take a seat, enquire as to the present situation, re-examine in order to ascertain that the indications for the proposed procedure were still present, explain the procedure to the patient and obtain consent. Dive straight in to discussing the pros and cons of including a local anaesthetic and the advantages or not of triamcinalone over hydrocortisone and a considerable number of marks will be lost.

9. Similarly, put down what you would actually do in the real world. Examiners are scathing of candidates who seem to work in practices where there are veritable armies of health visitors, social workers and community psychiatric nurses who seem qualified and willing to tackle every problem from child abuse to a major road traffic accident. Skills possessed by Primary Health Care Team members may be invaluable, possibly of some help or totally inappropriate. It makes sense to indicate to what extent their help would be helpful in your answer. However, if their involvement would not be appropriate their inclusion may actually lose you marks.

10. Abbreviations commonly used by candidates and by colleagues in their immediate vicinity may not be used or known to the examiner marking the paper. If the examiner cannot understand the answer no marks can be awarded. If abbreviations are required clarify them before repeating them in your answer e.g. myocardial infarction (MI). MI may then safely be repeated in the answer with the examiner aware that you mean myocardial infarction and not, for example, mitral incompetence.

11. Put the important facts or information down first. Less important information may well accrue marks but an answer indicating that thought has been given to the priority of the differential diagnosis, the most helpful therapeutic options or the difficulties to be tackled will attract more marks than one with a jumble of random thoughts.

12. Similarly, try to think in headings. There are often clear cut sections of an answer and it is again helpful to the marking examiner to structure your response in a neat, logical way. The use of 'skeletons' (see below) may help candidates who have difficulty in adjusting to the broadness of approach required so often in real general practice.

13. If an opportunity arises, mention any appropriate literature. Justification of relevant approaches in this way will attract high marks. Principal author, journal and year of publication would be more than satisfactory. Memorising journal volumes and page numbers would not seem to be a productive use of scarce revision time!

14. Finally, there are no marks awarded for writing 'etc.'. If there is more you can put down, put it down. If you can't think of anything else, don't waste the ink on etc.!

## Skeletons

Controversy rages over the use of skeletons in answering MEQs. Perhaps the key to understanding the MEQ is to think of providing answers as to what you *might* do. Many doctors are used to undergraduate and postgraduate medical examinations where there is usually only one 'right' answer–at least according to the examiners. In this examination the assessors deliberately set out to test what you *might* do rather than what you *would* do.

A GP's universal solution to every patient presenting with back pain might be an orthopaedic referral. Another GP might consider advice and analgesia, prescribing an anti-inflammatory agent, referring for physiotherapy/osteopathy/acupuncture, investigating with haematology, biochemistry or X-rays, an orthopaedic referral, a referral to a pain clinic, a referral to a psychologist, consideration of sick certification, liaising with the employers' medical service or the disabled resettlement office and so on. The ability to think broadly and offer alternative solutions to situations is part of quality general practice. Using skeletons regularly seems a good way for many GPs to get into this habit.

However, examiners are rightly critical of candidates who blithely answer each question using physical, psychological and social as their framework even when this is completely inappropriate. Consideration of the patient's knowledge, ideas and concerns, being able to consider a range of options and select the best, considering the management plan with the patient and being able to justify choices with reference to the literature are all high on the examiner's agenda. Candidates who apply a veneer of these attitudes by cramming heavily on technique may well score higher than they would otherwise do on the MEQ. However, this plan regularly falls apart later in the orals as these attributes are explored rigorously and with the candidate under more pressure.

Nevertheless, experience shows that a significant proportion of candidates who begin their preparation for the MRCGP require further practice in developing this broad, patient-centred approach. In many ways this is hardly surprising since the majority of candidates are vocational trainees, most of whom at this stage have had less than a year's experience of general practice. Working with colleagues on the half day release course should have given a wider perspective over the 3 years of vocational training. Unfortunately, the service commitment of the hospital jobs means that attendance is at best sporadic during the 2 years as Senior House Officer. Opportunities for formal study are rarely available and when they are, the energy to take advantage may be dissipated by too many busy nights on call.

One of the major justifications of having an MRCGP examination is that it is an incentive to study. We have found working at general practice problem cases using skeletons to be an effective way to steepen the learning curve of colleagues. Sometimes this enables them to appreciate for the first time the infinite potential of each general practice consultation, to consider other avenues of treatment and help, to consider their own and other people's feelings and to consider alternative courses of action when faced with very difficult but entirely realistic situations. We should welcome with open arms any educational method which helps us cope better with difficult areas of the job.

The examiners, however, are always right! Use the skeletons as an aid in studying – to appreciate the broad canvas general practice presents. Often with repetitive use they become ingrained so that it becomes second nature in a difficult consultation to select and use an appropriate skeleton as a mental checklist to cover aspects of the problem that would otherwise not be dealt with. Patients get a much better deal and doctors get more job satisfaction from this broad, patient-centred approach. If these attitudes and skills can begin to be appreciated and acquired during examination preparation the case for the MRCGP examination is greatly strengthened. It is a pity that such education is necessary so late in the period of professional training, but better late than never.

The skill is in selecting the appropriate skeleton and refining it to fit the problem presented. Of course, there are always problems that nothing could possibly prepare one for and in such a situation it's necessary to go back to basics and think things through as logically and calmly as possible!

Some examples of useful skeletons follow:

---

### THE INFINITE POTENTIAL OF THE CONSULTATION

*Time scale: now / soon / in the future*

- **History** particularly including the patient's ideas, concerns and expectations plus physical, psychological and social (money, housing, work, family, leisure and sex) factors as appropriate.
- **Examination**
- **Differential diagnosis**
- **Investigations**
- **Formulate management plan with patient +/– family**
- **Arrange help** family/ PHCT/ social services/ voluntary organisations
- **Refer**
- **Prescribe**
- **Anticipate problems in the future**
- **Prevention/health promotion**
- **Outline follow-up**
- **Liaise with other agencies**
- **Performance review**

---

NB: We work in the real world. Only a proportion of these areas could be covered in a single consultation even if they were all appropriate. Some might be worth looking at now, some later and some in the future – hence the timescale at the top. Most might be inappropriate in some situations and most entirely appropriate in others. The key is to be **selective** and work through the list logically.

---

### TREATMENT OPTIONS

- **Do nothing**
  - Follow-up at patient's discretion or formally arranged
- **Do something**
  - Discuss, bargain, counsel and advise.
  - Discuss other management options, obtain implied or informed consent
  - Prescribe drug and/or appliance
  - Arrange or carry out procedure
  - Arrange follow-up

---

The key point to appreciate from this skeleton is that there are almost always several options in any given situation. Some will almost always be appropriate, some hardly ever appropriate and some might be useful occasionally. Keeping this skeleton in mind can help broaden out approaches within consultations.

---

### REFERRAL OPTIONS

- **Within PHCT**
- **Secondary care**
  In-patient, out-patient, domiciliary visit, pathology and/or radiology, physiotherapy, day hospital, occupational therapy
  *Consider:*   NHS/Private local/regional/national implications of GP budget holding extra contractual referrals
- **Social services**
  social worker, day centre, meals on wheels, home helps, part III accommodation, orange disabled badge, welfare benefits, citizens advice
- **Other agencies**
  self help groups, voluntary groups, local and national hospices, Marie Curie Foundation, WRVS
- **Alternative therapies**

---

## CONSULTATION BEHAVIOUR

Particularly:

- **Explore**  patient's knowledge, ideas, concerns, expectations

- **Explain**  their symptoms and signs

- **Consider**  treatment options and advise patient

- **Consider**  patient's preference, involve patient in management plans

An alternative way of looking at the consultation is to divide it into:

- **Presenting  problems**
- **Continuing problems**
- **Help seeking behaviour**
- **Opportunistic health promotion**

Candidates generally would benefit by spending some time working at consultation dynamics and their own consultation techniques. A few skills learnt early in one's career can prevent a lot of heartache later on. For some doctors, learning consultation skills can mean the difference between job satisfaction and disillusionment. Read the literature. Use a video camera to record some consultations and analyse them with your trainer, course organiser or other resource person with some experience and expertise.

## IN A CONFLICT SITUATION

The options are:

- **Agree**
- **Disagree**
- **Refer**
- **Bargain**
- **Counsel**
- **Educate**

## GIVING BAD NEWS

- **Anxiety**  What are the patient's real fears and worries?

- **Knowledge**  How much does the patient know and understand already?

- **Explanation**  Covers diagnosis, prognosis, treatment and follow-up in terms the patient understands

- **Sympathy and Support**

## DEALING WITH ANGER

- Avoid confrontation
- Facilitate discussion
- Ventilate feelings
- Explore reasons for anger
- Consider referring or investigating

# Modified Essay Question Paper

## Instructions to candidates:

1. There are 10 questions in this paper.
2. Answers should be legible and concise. Total time allowed is 2 hours.
3. Answers should be written in the space provided. If more room is required use the reverse of the sheet.
4. The MEQ is a test of your practical approach and as such you could gain more for your management of the problem than for pure factual knowledge.
5. All questions carry equal marks; you are advised to work steadily through the paper and not delay too long on any one question.
6. Each page of the MEQ is marked independently. You should therefore answer each question specifically, even if this answer involves repetition of part of an earlier answer.

This paper is designed to provide realistic practice for examination candidates. Model answers are provided to indicate the sort of answers and areas the examiners would wish candidates to be considering. When studying this section candidates might find it helpful to consider the usefulness and the limitations of the skeletons mapped out in the MEQ seminar. Further progress can perhaps then be made by practising further MEQs under examination conditions from one of the several excellent examination preparation books. Another avenue worth exploring is to obtain past papers from the Royal College and in conjunction with others sitting the examination compare your performance to produce your own model answer. In the latter instance, help from a local trainer, course organiser, examiner or someone who has recently passed the examination would add an aura of street credibility.

*Page 1*

You are one of five full-time partners in a group practice located in a health centre with 10 000 patients. Each doctor looks after his/her personal list of patients. The practice is not fundholding. You have a full range of the usual ancillary and attached staff.

Your first patient of the morning is Fred Smith, aged 56. He attends for his third blood pressure reading. Two recent readings have been 165/100 and 160/90. Today's reading is 160/105. In the course of discussion Fred makes it clear that he does not wish to take tablets.

1. **How might you proceed with this consultation?**

Jane Taylor, a 35-year-old solicitor, attends for injection of her 'tennis elbow' (lateral epicondylitis).

2. **Give a step by step account of how you might proceed.**

You then see Janice and Michael who are residents at a local training centre for 27 young adult mentally handicapped patients. They are accompanied by their care helper. Janice and Michael have scabies.

**3. Discuss your management.**

Mrs Roberts, aged 45, is your next patient. She enquires about hormone replacement therapy because she has heard that it helps prevent osteoporosis.

**4. What factors would you take into account when considering your reply?**

Tracy Dwyer, aged 15, attends accompanied by her mother. She complains of a vaginal discharge. Mrs Dwyer remains in your consulting room whilst you examine Tracy in a separate examination room. Your practice nurse is present. Tracy tells you that she had sexual intercourse a week ago but asks that you do not tell her mother.

**5. Outline your management.**

Later, after surgery, you and your partners discuss a letter received from a patient who is a matron of a new nursing home for the elderly (the fifth similar nursing home recently built in your practice area). She asks that you and your partners take over the medical care of the residents.

**6.What issues would you wish to discuss with your partners before replying?**

You receive a message about Owen McIntyre, aged 11, who has advanced cerebral lymphoma. He has, at the request of his parents, been discharged from hospital for terminal care at home. His mother is a former district nurse and there is a brother aged 15 and a sister aged 18 both living at home. You decide to visit that afternoon.

**7. What areas will you need to cover in discussion with the McIntyre family?**

Owen McIntyre's clinical condition suggests to you that he will die within the next week or two.

**8. What will be your role following his death?**

At the monthly partners' business meeting one of your partners states that he refuses to complete the annual practice report.

**9. What may be the implications of this?**

**10. What may be the implications for general practice of information such as that contained in annual reports being available to FHSAs/ Health Boards?**

# The MEQ Model
Answers

# 1.

**Patient's ideas/concerns**
— Side effects?
— Denial of illness?
— Unaware of significance of raised blood pressure?

**Explore other risk factors**
— Smoking, family history, alcohol, weight, exercise, stress, diabetes

**Explanation by GP**
— Risks of hypertension
— Benefits of treatment
— Mention published evidence of benefit

**Examination and investigation**
— End-organ damage – e.g. fundoscopy, left ventricular hypertrophy, carotid bruits, peripheral pulses
— Investigations – e.g. test urine, ?MSU, U&E, ?random blood sugar, ?FBC

**Options/implications**
— No treatment – monitor BP
— Non-drug treatment – weight reduction, smoking, salt, exercise, relaxation, yoga
  Patient to consider pros and cons of treatment; either patient-initiated further discussion, definite follow-up appointment or simply opportunistic further care

## 2.

### Preparation
— Consent (usually implied, may be need for written in the future or in some circumstances)
— Explain procedure to patient in terms she understands
— Explore patient's ideas, concerns and expectations

### Procedure
— Localise site of maximum tenderness, confirming diagnosis
— Appropriate hygiene precautions
— Appropriate steroid +/− local anaesthetic
— Appropriate volume
— Patient comfortable and elbow supported
— Withdraw before inject
— Fanning injection

### Follow-up
— Immediate advice – appropriate rest period and analgesia
— When or if to return
— Advice re normal progress and complications (few and rare)

## 3.

### Immediate clinical management
— Method of treatment
— Choice of agent – pros and cons
— Consider strategy for other residents – ?appropriate at this time
— Prolonged close contact as mode of transmission + any other appropriate natural history of mite

### Follow-up
— Mention persistence of rash and itching after treatment
— ?Definite follow-up by self/practice or district nurse or other appropriate team member OR further appointment only if symptoms persist
— ?other residents/contacts may need information/review/support

### Communication
— With patients at their level including ideas, concerns, expectations
— With carers at their level including ideas, concerns, expectations
— Oral advice only or e.g. leaflets
— ? contact other GPs with patients in training centre

### Confidentiality
— Autonomy of disabled/communicating with carers and others
— Opportunistic health promotion
— Indication of prolonged close contact,?explore intimacy, contraception, sexually transmitted diseases

# 4.

**Patient's ideas, concerns, expectations**
— Amplify expectations of hormone replacement therapy
— Health beliefs, particularly re HRT, menopause
— Hidden agenda?

**Clinical aspects**
— Current health problems – especially hot flushes, insomnia, vaginal dryness
— Current gynaecological state – still menstruating? If postmenopausal with a uterus does she accept restarting periods and risk of D&C being necessary if irregular bleeding occurs?
— Past medical history – especially breast or uterine malignancy and any thromboembolic problem
— Family history

**Explanation**
— Values of HRT including different therapeutic approaches and length of treatment course thought to be required for osteoporosis prevention
— Risks of HRT
— All in terms patient understands. Options/implications/choice
— Necessity for follow-up and information re symptoms of potential side effects

**Ethical issues**
— Discussion re use of resources (medical time, finance) versus potential savings (morbidity, mortality and finance)

**Opportunistic health promotion**
— Blood pressure, smear, weight, smoking, urine, alcohol, exercise, lifestyle

**Practice organisation**
— Discussion re delegation to practice nurse +/– clinic with protocol

## 5.

**Clinical**
— Steady/casual boyfriend
— Need for accurate diagnosis re discharge – investigate in surgery or refer STD?
— Treat discharge blind or wait for result of investigations?
— Hidden agenda – explore for hints of sexual abuse/assault
— Possibility of pregnancy

**Ideas, concerns, expectations**
— Tracy is a minor
— Requires confidentiality and respect for autonomy
— Explore fears
— Explore feelings
— Explore contraceptive needs

**Further management**
— Anything clinically appropriate for discharge or contraception
— Facilitate discussion with mother/ family if appropriate
— Discretion
— Consider further emotional support required
— Safe sex

## 6.

**Practical points**
— May be only practice in the area – in which case have no choice but  perhaps have an influence over the home's policies re e.g. calls, prescribing
— If other local practices, patients may wish to retain present GP and GPs may wish to retain patient.
— A blanket refusal may offend matron who is a patient of the practice.
— Patients should retain personal autonomy.
— NHS reforms advocate greater patient choice.
— What is the practice policy re making potentially contentious decisions?

**Factors influencing decision**
— Additional income, more work, current practice age-sex distribution, special interest/expertise amongst partners, admission policy of home re level of disability cared for, ?private retainer fee envisaged from home to practice for non-NHS services

**Practice organisation**
— Share list/workload or all to one partner?
— ?rearrange/drop other commitments
— ?regular visit/'ward round'
— Prescription organisation/notes
— Agree protocols for minor illnesses and requests for visits
— Discuss with other members of PHCT

**Matters to clarify with home**
— Working practices/protocols (see above)
— Staff experience/training
— Standards of care
— Health Authority approval
— Non-NHS fee? (see above)

**Future implications**
— Local policy re homes?
— Liaise with FHSA, local authority, Health Authority, social services, other practices?
— Demographic inevitability

## 7.

**Current state of knowledge**
— Owen, parents, siblings
— Other members of family (close and distant)
— Friends of Owen, of parents, of siblings.
— is everyone aware of diagnosis and prognosis. Can we facilitate this?
— what are the fears, concerns and expectations?
— are they aware of the local support and help available?
— feelings/distress/preparing and pre-bereavement counselling if appropriate at this stage (may not be on a first visit)
— encourage realistic expectations (may be too low or too high)

**Medical commitment**
— Personal availability whenever possible, consistent with personal and family needs – liaise with receptionists and family to facilitate this
— Arrangements for contacting in and out of hours
— Empathy

**Coping plans**
— Pain and symptom control
— Nursing plans
— Liaison with community nurses, McMillan nurses, hospice and other local services as appropriate
— Spiritual support from local church if appropriate

**Assess family resources**
— Physical: home, bedroom/toilet, extended support available from family/ friends to share nursing burden if necessary
— Psychological: Owen, parents and siblings' current feelings
— Social:  family integration and support, facilitate appropriate current and future normality as far as possible for all concerned
— Benefits – ?attendance allowance

**Future support**
— Emphasise availability, support and empathy for physical, psychological and social problems

## 8.

### Immediate/soon after death
— Confirm death
— Death +/– cremation forms, liaison with undertaker, second doctor for cremation forms, ?vicar/priest
— Notify PHCT, hospital team(s) and other caring agencies involved
— Note in parents' and siblings' medical records for future reference

### Initial support
— Praise/support nursing care provided
— Share feelings/facilitate any initial feelings of disbelief, guilt or anger and reassure re these
— Explain normal bereavement reaction
— Consider short term sedation (but avoid medicalising normal grief reaction)

### Medium term
— Follow-up visit
— Advice on returning to normal pattern of life – school and work
— Ventilate feelings/encourage further discussions re Owen between family members
— Assure of continuing availability of these discussions or other problems
— Monitor progress of grief reaction
— Support may also be required for other carers or self

### Long term
— Death of a child from cancer may have on-going effects on family, friends and community
— Be aware of anniversaries, be aware of  unresolved grief reactions

**9.**

### Clarification
— Does the partner simply wish someone else to take on this task *or*
— Is this a statement indicating non-cooperation 'on any grounds'?
— Why now? Are there problems with the practice, partners, personally or at home?

### Implications for practice and partners
— Partnership or individual may be in breach of  terms of service if annual report not completed
— FHSA may be unable to assess allocation of resources e.g. staff bids, improvement grant applications, computer reimbursement without some indication of practice activities and plans
— Ideally relationship between practice and FHSA should be cooperation – this could sour it
— Another partner may well have to take on this task instead – an additional burden for him/her
— Discord and partnership difficulties may affect  morale of partners and practice

### Implications for partner
— Stress/burnout/particular current difficulty?
— Who can help? – partners, staff, family, friends, own GP?
— Is there evidence of problems in other areas?  These may not be apparent if the partnership operates strict personal lists
— Do we just need to talk about things more?
— Have the doctors been so busy looking after the patients that they don't look after each other?

### Implications for patients
— Partner may have more time for them if not doing annual report
— Short term may therefore benefit but medium term may suffer if practice resources threatened

### Implications for staff
— May be under threat if resources from FHSA threatened
— May be affected if partner/partnership has problems

# 10.

## For the practice

— Positive
— Encourage clinical audit/setting practice standards
— Encourage administrative/financial audit
— Encourage discussion and planning for the future
— Publicity?
— Negative
— Data inadequate for satisfactory conclusions to be drawn
— Outside body being judgemental/imposing standards inappropriately
— Feeling of loss of independence/practice autonomy

## For the patients

— Increases patient autonomy/choice (but poor evidence that many are good 'choosers')
— May lead to better clinical care, better planning and better practice administration resulting in more efficient service
— Doctors and practice staff may spend time on preparing statistics and be less available for clinical care
— Care required by practice to protect patient confidentiality
— Standards imposed from outside may, in a worst case scenario, lead to the removal of valued and appropriate patient services

## Administration/finance

— Better budgetary control within practice
— Potentially more appropriate use of NHS resources and better planning for implementing expansion/changes in services, premises, staff, training
— Potential to demonstrate some markers of 'good practice'

# ■ 5
# The Critical Reading Question Paper

■ Format
■ Content
■ Technique
■ CRQ Practice Paper
  — Questions
  — Answers

The Critical Reading Question paper replaced the Practice Topic Question paper in the autumn of 1990.

The new paper's title has been given the acronym of CRQ, and the wisdom of the examiners who recommended changing the title from the original Critical Reading and Audit Paper has therefore been amply demonstrated!

Most candidates when first faced with the prospect of the CRQ paper are apprehensive. Criticising a published paper is not an everyday activity for most young GPs. However, actually assessing a paper is only one part out of (usually) eight in this 2 hour paper – and even that is just a matter of knowing what to look for combined with a little common sense. As for the other eight parts, the candidate who reads widely and critically will do well. Those that do not will have difficulties.

## Format

The candidate has 2 hours to answer (usually) three questions which are further divided into parts. Unless advised otherwise an answer in the form of expanded notes would be expected. Another 15 minutes or so are provided for candidates to read the presented material. All three questions in their parts are contained in a booklet of a similar format to the MEQ paper.

Each *part* carries equal marks. It is therefore VITAL to allocate an equal amount of time to each part. As in the MEQ paper, the marking schedules will ensure that most marks are gained for the most important points. These will be made early on in an answer and candidates who spend a long time making erudite but perhaps irrelevant points will find it difficult to accumulate further marks on that question. Running over time will certainly result in a candidate having less time to answer another part of the paper, and perhaps not answering a question or part question well enough to accumulate the 'soft' basic marks that should at least ensure achieving the level of a pass. Running out of time and not answering part of the paper at all is one of the greatest sins any examination candidate can commit – no answer means zero marks and however well the other parts are answered the few extra marks gained will not compensate when the mark for the whole paper is totalled.

The stated aim of the CRQ paper is to assess the candidate's ability to understand, summarise and evaluate published papers and written material encountered in general practice, together with the ability to apply appropriately what has been read to the setting of modern British primary care.

# Content

### Question 1

In Question 1 candidates will be given a published paper from an established general medical journal relevant to British general practice. This will be presented without the abstract since the question will test the ability to:

---

   (i)  recognise the main issues raised
   (ii)  comment where appropriate on the design of the study and
   (iii)  discuss the implications and practical application of the results to general practice.

---

Given practice at the technique, the first and third parts should present little difficulty. Most doctors familiar with reading the BMJ and the BJGP regularly should have no difficulty providing the examiners with a simple precis of a paper. The structured abstract provides a ready made framework:

---

— objective
— design
— setting
— subjects
— main outcome measures
— results
— conclusions

---

Experience and understanding of the organisation of British general practices will mean that candidates can rapidly put together an answer relating to implications and practical applica-

tions. Remember not to be too narrow and doctor-centred – consider the effects on:

---

— personal patient management
— practice policies
— practice organisation
— practice finance
— the work of primary health care team members
— referral patterns
— prescribing costs
— workload of consultants and other hospital staff
— district resources e.g. pathology
— own workload/free time
— society as a whole

---

With regard to critical appraisal of study design, the RCGPs recommended reading list for the CRQ contains advice and help. The following notes provide a framework:

1. The paper presented should contain:

---

— an accurate title
— a reproducible method
— clear-cut sections
— discernible raw data
— credible results
— justifiable conclusions
— correct references.

---

2. Descriptive reports, audit and epidemiological studies:

---

— should have a clear aim
— have the potential to produce a significant clinical and/or organisational change
— should define clearly and appropriately exclusions and withdrawals
— withdrawals should account for less than 10% of the total
— should be analysed correctly and fully.

---

3. A randomised controlled trial in addition to the above:

---

— must be ethical
— must be randomised by a proper blind

method
— should be prospective
— exclusions must take place before randomisation
— should have defined and appropriate treatment regimens, contemporary control groups and end-points.

4. All papers:

— should specify the sample under study
— have strict criteria for diagnosis
— detail alternative risk factors which might influence the study e.g. age, smoking, social class, race, presence of coexistent morbidity
— use statistical results correctly.

In practical terms, criticising a paper means looking at the good points of the study and then describing some of the questionable aspects of the study. Remember that there will be perhaps 10 or 15 minutes to make the salient points the examiners are looking for. It is highly unlikely, therefore, that the examiners will expect MRCGP candidates to carry out an expert statistical analysis of a complicated paper in the examination. Such activities take full-time statisticians many hours.

It is much more likely that candidates will be looking for:

— errors in sample groups or questionnaire design
— a failure to describe the method clearly
— problems with alternative risk factors, exclusions and withdrawals
— end-points and diagnostic definitions unclear.

Candidates are often over-awed by the prospect of what is, in the end, a pretty straightforward task once one knows what to do and where to look for the common questionable areas.

## Question 2

It is likely that Question 2 will be in parts since it is designed to test familiarity with published literature in areas of current interest in general practice. Most marks will not be given for listing references but for demonstrating a broad grasp of the issues involved.

If there are three parts to this question the candidate only has a little over 10 minutes to get the relevant facts down on paper to get adequate marks on each part. Fine detail is unlikely to be rewarded. The picture should be painted with a broad brush. Try again to think of the options, implications and choice under as wide a range of headings as is appropriate. The same groups involved when answering the implications in Question 1 should be considered.

Familiarity with other sections of this book and structured reading, particularly of the last 2 years' issues of the BMJ and BJGP should ensure good marks. The creation of a key word index as described earlier seems the logical way to prepare.

## Question 3

This is an interesting innovation of a technique used extensively in vocational training. The candidate will be presented with written material commonly encountered in general practice. This might be a letter, a practice protocol, a practice report, a piece of general practice audit, advertising material or, indeed, anything else appropriate. It would seem prudent to be prepared for a surprise! Candidates are expected to analyse the practical implications of the presented material to their work as general practitioners.

Once again it would seem likely that candidates will gain an adequate number of marks if they adopt the policy of considering a broad range of alternative responses, as well as the implications for the patient, their family, society as a whole, the doctor and as wide a range of colleagues as possible. Narrowing down onto just one or two doctor implications or responses is likely to result in relatively few marks being gained. Obtaining some past papers, familiarising oneself with the likely type of material and practising in a group setting if possible are likely to be particularly beneficial for Question 3.

# Technique

Candidates should use exactly the same technique described in detail in the MEQ section. In summary:

1. Write your name on the front of the booklet and check the instructions for any surprise changes.
2. Check each page has your candidate's number.
3. Divide the time available equally between the parts.
4. Read the questions before you read the presented material – you will then be reading with an eye to the questions you have to answer.
5. Write legibly in note form.
6. Carry information backwards and forwards onto separate sheets appropriately as again the sheets are marked by different examiners.
7. Write 'PTO' boldly if you turn over the page.
8. Answer the question posed and only the question posed – read the question carefully.
9. State the obvious.
10. Be realistic – we all have to work in the real world and not in a utopian dream.
11. Be careful with abbreviations.

# Critical Reading Question Paper

**Instructions to candidates:**

1. You are advised to read the relevant questions before reading the presented material.
2. There are eight question parts in this paper. Each part carries equal marks.
3. Answers should be in expanded note form.
4. Each page is marked by a different examiner. You should therefore give a complete answer to each question even if this involves repetition of part of an earlier answer.
5. Answers should be written in the space provided.
6. In question 2 you will gain marks when mentioning current literature by describing its contribution to the arguments which you are presenting and, where appropriate, commenting on its credibility. If possible you should indicate the source and approximate year of publication. Merely listing references will not suffice. The majority of marks are awarded for clearly stating the current views on the topic.

This paper is presented to candidates with the aim of providing them with realistic examination practice. Maximum benefit from this exercise will be obtained if the candidate arranges for, say, the local librarian or practice secretary to copy the following paper and blank out the abstract. The paper should then be presented to the candidate in a sealed envelope. To practise under realistic conditions, remember that this paper is 2 hours long, with an additional 15 minutes for reading the presented material.

The paper used in this practice paper is:
Salisbury C J 1989 How do people choose their doctor? BMJ 299: 608–610

Salisbury C J 1989 How do people choose their doctor? BMJ 299: 608–610

**Question 1A**
**Write an abstract for this paper.**

Salisbury C J 1989 How do people choose their doctor? BMJ 299: 608–610

**Question 1B**
**Comment on the study design.  List the ways in which the response rate might have been improved.**

*Page 3*

Salisbury C J 1989 How do people choose their doctor? BMJ 299: 608–610

**Question 1C**
**Assuming that the findings are supported by further studies what are the implications for general practice?**

**Question 2A**
**Discuss recent evidence supporting longer consultations in general practice.**

**Question 2B**
**Discuss the evidence concerning the role of antibiotics in treating otitis media in children.**

**Question 2C**
**Discuss current views on intrapartum obstetric care by general practitioners.**

Reference: Page 9 – Letter from consultant

**Question 3A**
**What are the issues raised by this letter from the consultant gynaecologist?**

The MRCGP Workbook

Reference: Page 9 – Letter from consultant

**Question 3B**
**What are your options for management? Give reasons for your favoured approach.**

ANYTOWN  HEALTH AUTHORITY

ANYTOWN DISTRICT HOSPITAL

Dr D. Smith
The Health Centre
Anytown

Dear David,

Re:  Jane Doe, 31 High Street, Anytown

This patient came to see me today without a letter. She is only 15 years old and has had four sexual partners in her short life. She attended the Family Planning Clinic and saw a lady doctor with glasses but was refused contraception before she became pregnant. I think this was a TERRIBLE mistake which ought not to happen nowadays. She is 8 weeks pregnant. I am prepared to do a termination of pregnancy on her but we have the problem that she is under 16 and we need someone to sign the consent form. Could you think about this one because she refuses absolutely to tell her mother and father. She says that if she tells her parents that she is pregnant, she will be thrown out of the house.

Yours sincerely,

Frank

Mr F. Zebedee   FRCOG
Consultant Gynaecologist/Obstetrician

PS Perhaps you could tell the Family Planning Doctor of my comments.

# CRQ Model Answers

# Question 1A

## Objective
— To study how people find out about their doctors, why they change practices and what factors influence their choice of general practitioner.

## Design
— Postal questionnaire, preceded by a pilot. A follow-up questionnaire was sent to non-responders and a further shorter questionnaire to persisting non-responders.

## Setting
— General practice.

## Subjects
— 791 people registering with five practices over an 8 week period in Jan–Mar 1989. These represented 447 individuals or family units.

## Results
— 65% response rate to full questionnaire, increasing to 72% with replies to shorter reminder questionnaire.
— 67% of responders chose the practice either because it was the nearest or following a recommendation. A further 16% registered because another member of the family was registered there. Only 4% of those registering did any comparison of practices beforehand.
— 83% of those registering did so following a change of address. However, only 58% registered within 4 months of their move, 18% waited over 12 months before registering and 47% waited until they were ill.
— Only 5% registered because they were dissatisfied with their existing practice; a further 5% registered because the new surgery was more convenient.
— 47% heard about the practice from recommendations and 33% through seeing the surgery buildings.
— 40% of those registering knew nothing about the practice before registering. 24% had gathered information only from friends or relatives.
— Patients rated a friendly doctor, helpful receptionists, an efficient appointments system, convenient surgery hours and preventative medicine as important desirable attributes of a practice. However, there is no evidence that they used this information when selecting a practice.

## Conclusion
— There is remarkably little evidence of consumerism operating in the way people choose their doctor.

# Question 1B

### Points in favour of the method
— Adequate response rate
— Use of pilot questionnaire(s)
— No social or age bias
— Adequate sample size
— Questionnaire design used open and closed questions

### Questionable aspects of method
— Shorter questionnaire as second reminder means two questionnaires used
— Origin of questionnaire may be seen by responders as important and may influence results
— No. of questions in questionnaire important in response
— Sex bias in responders
— Distribution between five practices is not stated

### Response rate might be improved by:
— Pre-paid envelope for reply
— Personal interviews
— Approach from doctor – letter/telephone/in person
— Incentives for responders
— Distribution of questionnaires at the time of registration

## Question 1C

— There is little evidence to suggest patients choose their doctor on an informed basis. Consumers, therefore, cannot be relied upon to reward good doctors.

— When asked for desirable practice attributes, patients rate approachability, accessibility and preventative medicine highest.

— Patient demands and needs are not necessarily the same.

— A friendly consulting style and an efficient appointments system are better use of time and energy for a practice than 'advertising'.

— Public awareness of the need to register with a doctor after a house move, and availability of practice leaflets and other sources of  information will need to be increased before patients even begin to exercise some discrimination in their choice of doctor.

## Question 2A

Consultation length has increased from 6–7 minutes 20 years ago to 8–9 minutes at the present. Is this important?

Wilson (1992 BMJ) showed that recording of blood pressure, smoking, alcohol consumption and advice about immunisation were all greater in surgeries booked at 10 minute intervals, when compared with the doctor's usual rate of 6 minute intervals. However, the actual consultation length only increased from 7 to 8 minutes.

Howie (1991 JRCGP) showed that longer consultations meant more psychological problems were tackled, more long term health problems were dealt with and more health promotion was undertaken.

Howie's department has also shown in two further papers in 1991 and 1992 in the BJGP that longer booking intervals mean shorter time for patients in the waiting room and less stress for doctors, particularly those practising in a patient-centred style.

An innovative approach has been tried where patients choose their own appointment length (Lowenthal & Bingham 1987 BJGP). This was reported as being very successful but has probably not been widely adopted due to general practice having undergone considerable changes associated with the 1990 Contract and the NHS reforms – one further major change in appointment systems is not easily accommodated in such circumstances.

## Question 2B

Most general practitioners in Great Britain still treat otitis media with antibiotics. Many parents see children with earache as a medical emergency necessitating urgent treatment in or out of hours. However, general practitioners in other countries see things differently – in Holland antibiotics are prescribed much less frequently for otitis media – and evidence is still accumulating that less frequent prescribing may be appropriate.

Burke (1991 BMJ) showed in a controlled trial that the outcome was the same whether analgesia only or antibiotics were prescribed. However, pain relief was achieved more quickly in the antibiotic group. This paper was unfortunately flawed by the poor definition of exclusions and the perhaps inevitable selection of arbitrary medium and long term assessment points.

Browning & Bain (1990 BMJ) also showed that antibiotics may not influence outcome.

The different international picture was described by Froom (1990 BMJ).

Perhaps at the present a reasonable policy would be to look critically at each middle ear infection rather than prescribing antibiotics as almost an automatic reflex. Encouragement of early use of analgesia by parents may obviate the need for some prescriptions or even consultations. Advice and analgesia with early review may also be an acceptable management plan. Persistent pyrexia, pain and systemic upset despite symptomatic treatment still probably warrant antibiotics – though perhaps not with a 30 minute history at 3 a.m.

# Question 2C

There has been historical criticism of the quality of general practice intrapartum care. Most of this has come from hospital consultants. Marsh (1977 BMJ) and Klein (1983 BJObs&Gyn), however, showed impressive safety records as good or better than consultant units. Tew (1985 JRCGP) showed a record better than consultant units even after allowances are made for the high-risk cases booked in consultant units.

The trend continues in recent times with Bryce et al and Sangala et al (both 1990 BMJ) as hospital specialists criticise GPs with a host of other papers (Street, Ford et al and Campbell et al – all 1991 BMJ) showing adequate safety.

Why then do relatively few GPs undertake intrapartum GP obstetrics? Consumer choice supports GP obstetrics, isolated units mean there is sometimes no available alternative for geographical reasons and home confinements are still requested by some patients.

Two recent papers shed some light on the attitudes of GPs by looking at GP trainees. Despite training conferring skills, confidence was lacking. GP obstetrics was regarded as a high risk activity (Smith 1991 and 1992 BMJ).

The present workload of general practitioners, particularly the increasing out-of-hours workload, changing working patterns with cooperatives and deputising services, closure of isolated maternity units and still poor financial rewards all mean that GP intrapartum obstetrics remains a minority activity.

# Question 3A

**Issues raised are:**

— no referral letter. Gone astray?, self-referred?, concealed?
— multiple sexual partners in a teenager confers health risks STD, cervical dysplasia, HIV
— contraception required – but patient is a minor
— consent required – patient is a minor
— patient autonomy and confidentiality need to be respected
— relationship between patient, parents and doctor needs to be preserved
— relationship between GP, consultant and patient needs to be addressed
— relationship between GP, consultant and FP doctor needs to be considered
— patient needs access to GP and vice versa.

# Question 3B

## 1. Seek advice

— Likely sources are partners, medical defense society – particularly re consent and contraception.

— Other sources are the consultant, BMA, informal local network – e.g. RCGP faculty.

## 2. Check with notes

— Patient's and parents' may yield useful information and background.

— Check re-referral letter.

## 3. Make contact with patient

— May be difficult but need to preserve confidentiality.

— School nurse, health visitor, practice or district nurse or even school may be appropriate and confidential intermediary.

— Need to set aside sufficient time with patient for potentially long, difficult consultation.

## 4. Consultation

— Establish rapport.

— Establish patient's understanding of current situation.

— Offer empathy/sympathy – very difficult situation for her.

— Explore patient's ideas, expectations, concerns and wishes.

— Encourage disclosure to parents.

— Arrange follow-up appointment at which to make definitive management plan.

## 5. Management plan

— Appropriate plan constructed including patient autonomy and consent issues, preferably with parental involvement and agreement of all parties.

## 6. Follow-up

— Including contraception and safe sex advice. Consider STD screening and cervical cytology.

— ? further consultation with parents to debrief/support.

## 7. Communication with professional colleagues

— Sort out issue of missing letter.

— If appropriate, discuss case with consultant and FP doctor in non-confrontational way and with patient's permission.

## 8. 'Self' care

— Difficult case – may have been a problem for self and other members of team involved. Do we need to talk?

# 6

# Revision Topics and Relevant Papers

This section is designed to:

1. Illustrate the sort of document that diligent MRCGP examination candidates might produce from reading the last 2 years' issues of the BMJ and BJGP as required by the CRQ paper.

2. Provide candidates with some short cuts into some of the medical literature that may be particularly relevant to general practice.

It must be emphasised that original papers need to be consulted to provide a proper and full sense of perspective – simply reading the following pages and believing that one has suddenly become knowledgeable about the literature of general practice will lead to disaster. If only life was as easy as that.

Where appropriate, some of the references quoted here are deliberately a few years old and may at first sight seem out of date. However, they are actually included either to give an appropriate sense of the way present understanding of a particular problem has evolved, or because the paper was or still is a classic in its subject area.

Key questions are highlighted to make candidates *think* about the subject as they read the original papers.

The amount of reading required of MRCGP candidates makes for better general practitioners. It actually becomes very rewarding for general practitioners to be able to discuss sensitively a management dilemma with a patient secure in the knowledge that the core information one is giving the patient is absolutely accurate and up to date. What might previously have been difficult consultations because of one's own uncertainty can be transformed simply by examination preparation.

## Screening the elderly

### Key questions

– How do you organise the over 75 screening programme?

– What is the purpose of this activity?

– What are the advantages of screening the over 75s?

– What are the disadvantages of screening the over 75s?

– Has the practice audited its elderly screening programme?

– Does the practice programme stand up to scrutiny?

– Does the practice programme require modification?

– Does the national programme need modification?

1. **The elderly as under consulters: a critical appraisal**

   Taylor R, Ford G 1983 JRCGP 33: 699–705

2. **Low levels of ill health among elderly non-consulters in general practice**

   Ebrahim S, Hedley R, Sheldon M 1984 BMJ 289: 1273–1275

Both of these studies showed that few new medical problems were identified by the screening programmes...

3. **Consequences of assessment and intervention among elderly people: a three year randomised controlled trial**

   Hendrikson C, Lund E, Stromgard E 1984 BMJ 289: 1522–1524

4. **A randomised controlled trial of geriatric screening and surveillance in general practice**

   Tulloch A J, Moore V 1979 JRCGP 29: 733–742

... but controlled trials have shown fewer days in nursing homes and hospital and reduced mortality in the intervention groups.

5. **Screening the elderly in the community: controlled trial of dependency surveillance using a questionnaire administered by volunteers**

Carpenter G I, Demopoulos G R 1990 BMJ 300: 1253–1256

No difference in mortality or in morbidity scores between intervention and control group. More falls in the control group who spent more time in institutional care. However, the intervention group spent more time in hospital and they received community support services sooner than the control group. The scheme was popular with the majority of those studied.

6. **Age, pattern of consultation and functional disability in elderly patients in one general practice**

   Hall R G P, Channing D M 1990 BMJ 301: 424–428

Functional disability is easily assessed by adding up the number of surgery attendances and home visits – more GP involvement = greater disability. Put more simply, GPs already know most if not all the medical problems of the elderly.

7. **Screening elderly patients**

   McLennan W J 1990 BMJ 300: 694–695

Useful overview from a Professor of Geriatric Medicine

8. **Assessment of elderly people in general practice**

   1. **Social circumstances and mental state**

   2. **Functional abilities and medical problems**

      Iliffe S et al 1991 BJGP 41: 9–15

These are two comprehensive papers. 22% had evidence of depression, 15% had cognitive impairment, 18% were incontinent of urine and 6% were incontinent of faeces (only 1 patient out of the 239 with incontinence had laundry service support). The setting for the study was North and North-West London.

9. **Case finding in elderly people: validation of a postal questionnaire**

   Bowns I et al 1991 BJGP 41: 100–104

The prior use of a postal questionnaire reduced the need to visit and assess by between a third and a half and reliably detected those at greatest risk. This has obvious resource implications.

## 10. Can health visitors prevent fractures in elderly people?

Vetter N J, Lewis P A, Ford D 1992 BMJ 304: 888–890

Despite an approach involving assessing and correcting nutritional deficiencies, alcohol and smoking advice, assessment of medical conditions and medication, assessment and correction of environmental hazards in the home and improvement of fitness over a 4 year programme there was no effect on the incidence of fractures. Tremendous commitment of resources for no benefit.

## 11. Screening elderly people: a review of the literature in the light of the new general practitioner contract

Perkins E R 1991 BJGP   41: 382–385

This wide-ranging review article also concludes that the 1990 contract version of elderly screening does not have value but the literature reveals that there may be some benefits of screening the elderly that are worth further enquiry.

## 12. Health checks on patients 75 years and over in Nottinghamshire after the new GP contract

Brown K et al 1992 BMJ   305: 619–621

## 13. Assessment of patients aged over 75 in general practice

Tremellen J 1992 BMJ   305: 621–624

## 14. Health checks for people over 75 – the doubts persist

Harris A 1992 BMJ Editorial 305: 599–600

These studies show that the screening is being applied in a variety of ways with a variety of personnel. Doubts continue to exist as to whether the present wide-ranging annual check is the best way of utilising resources. Harris suggests a more focused check at 75 and 78 years looking specifically at detecting hypertension

and treatable functional disabilities – hearing and foot problems in particular. There has been little or no work done to determine whether the provision of resources is adequate to meet discovered functional disabilities.

## 15. Are elderly people living alone an at risk group?

Iliffe S et al  1992 BMJ 305: 1001–1004

No – so any revision of arrangements targeting this group would not be appropriate.

## 16. Randomised trial of case finding and surveillance of elderly people at home

Pathy M S J et al 1992 Lancet 340: 890–893

Recognising the practical difficulties and resource implications of comprehensive screening of the elderly by home visits, this approach involved a postal questionnaire being sent to a random sample of patients over 65. Where potential health problems were revealed they were followed up. Three years later there were fewer deaths, more surgery consultations and fewer home visits in the intervention group. The number of hospital admissions was not altered by intervention although length of stay in the intervention group was shorter.

## 17. Are preventative visits to the over 75s of any value?

Williams E I   Update  15th December 1992, p1035–1039

Professor Williams seems overall to be in favour of screening the over 75s. Even so he lists 10 advantages of screening and nine disadvantages.

## 18. Elderly people's views of an annual screening assessment

McIntosh I B, Power K G 1993 BJGP 43: 189–192

One of the worries about preventative medicine is that the screening itself may induce anxiety in those being screened. If this is the case, in programmes with a low detection rate it may be debatable whether the advantages of the programme outweigh the harm caused by the screening. This paper is reassuring about the anxiety level induced by screening the elderly, although the results may not be generally applicable since the assessment programme used in this study extended considerably beyond contractual obligations.

# Out-of-hours calls

## Key questions

- What does a GP's contract say about 24 hour responsibility?

- Is this still appropriate more that 40 years after the first NHS contract?

- What is happening to the practice night visiting rate? Why?

- What is happening to the national night visiting rate? Why?

- What do you feel about the use of deputising services?

- How does a GP Cooperative differ from a deputising service?

- How do you cope after a busy weekend on call with Monday's normal workload?

- Given a free hand, would you reorganise out-of-hours care? How?

## 1. On-call

Knox J D E 1989 Practical guides for general practice – 9. Oxford Medical Publications

A classic. A little basic perhaps but full of useful suggestions which guide the reader towards good practice without preaching. Only 64 pages including five appendices.

## 2. Effects of sleep disruption on cognitive performance and mood in medical house officers

Deary I, Tait R 1987 BMJ 295: 1513–1516

The authors conclude that though loss of sleep and long hours of work have an effect on memory and mood, the individual differences among doctors are the main source of the variance in the performance of tasks. This begs the question as to whether the man on the Clapham omnibus is appropriately looked after by a tired and irritable GP who has just had a busy and difficult weekend on call and who can't remember what examination he was going to perform before the telephone rang and interrupted the consultation. Patient's prescriptions may be correctly written but how much warmth and empathy can one drag up by 6 p.m. Monday after a weekend on-call?

## 3. Variations in GP night visiting rates: medical organisation and consumer demand

Buxton M J, Klein R E, Sayers J 1977 BMJ 1, 827–830

A considerable increase in claims over a 10 year period, with considerable differences between areas in night visit fees claimed. The factors most strongly associated with the higher rates were deputising services and the proportion of social class V in the population.

## 4. Provision of first contact care out of hours in four urban areas in England

Williams B T, Dixon R A, Nicholl J P 1985 BMJ 291: 1689–1692

In a typical 2 week period in 1984, 40% of first contacts out of hours were with hospital A&E departments, 25% with deputising services and 33% with the patients' own practice.

## 5. Patient satisfaction with general practitioner deputising services

Dixon R A, Williams B T 1988 BMJ 297: 1519–1522

A high proportion of patients were satisfied with the deputising service they received.

## 6. A study of telephone advice in managing out of hours calls

Marsh G N, Horne R A, Channing D M 1987 JRCGP 37: 301–304

59% of calls were managed with telephone advice with no apparent detriment to patients' health.

### 7. Out of hours workload of a surburban general practice: deprivation or expectation

Pitts J, Whitby M 1990 BMJ 300: 1113–1115

A high contact rate in a relatively affluent area, a considerable proportion from the casualty department of the local cottage hospital. 44% handled by telephone advice. The problems generated by this volume of out of hours work are discussed. The authors believe that patients now expect a 24 hours general medical service.
See also BMJ letters, 9 June 1990; 300: 1527.

### 8. Out of hours work in general practice

Iliffe S, Haug U 1991 BMJ 303: 1584–1586

An extremely cogent argument is put together by the authors who summarise the difficulties in providing appropriate care, avoiding exhausted doctors and coping with increasing demand. Their solution is a redefined GP contract covering a 17 hour day with deputising services funded by health authorities based on the existing network of A&E departments, health centres and clinics. 'If it is possible for a large supermarket chain to place an outlet within 10 miles of 90% of the population, then the biggest employer in western Europe should be able to do the same or better.' Once we get to that stage, do we then move on to a salaried service?

### 9. Visiting through the night

Salisbury C 1993 BMJ 306: 762–764

### Night visits and general practice

Williams B T 1993 BMJ Editorial 306: 734–735

This paper and an accompanying editorial describe and discuss the accelerating trend in the number of night visits. Chris Salisbury also suggests a revision of GP contracts, with the hours between midnight and 7a.m. the responsibility of FHSAs. If the trend described continues no one will be able to cope without some respite. Are patients benefiting? Are the calls appropriate?

# GP Obstetrics

### Key questions

– How do you feel about GP intrapartum care?

– What is the GP's role in obstetrics?

– Is GP obstetrics safe?

– Is GP obstetrics important?

– Why do so few GPs undertake home deliveries? Should GPs be prepared to do more?

– What do you say to someone who requests a home confinement?

– What are the choices for delivery and care in your district?

– Why do so few GPs get involved with intrapartum care?

– Given a choice, how would you organise intrapartum care for your patients? Justify your plan.

### 1. Critical appraisal of domiciliary obstetric and neonatal practice

Cox C A et al 1976 BMJ 1: 84

### 2. The general practitioner's role in the management of labour

Curzon P 1976 BMJ 2: 1433

### 3. Chamberlain G 1977 (letter) BMJ 1: 168

Continuing the trend of the preceding 10 years, these papers try to show how inadvisable it is for GPs to undertake obstetric care, particularly intrapartum care.

### 4. Home deliveries

Reilly W J 21 April 1979 Personal view. BMJ 1979; 3: 1077

### 5. Domiciliary obstetrics

Russell J K 1979 BMJ 2: 377–378

Cautionary tales from days past – a steady undermining of confidence in skills being practised in conditions not appropriate to modern standards of care and safety.

### 6. Obstetric audit in general practice

Marsh G N 1977 BMJ 2: 1004–1006

Going against the trend at the time, Geoffrey Marsh showed the way with carefully selected cases and a committed team approach producing an impressive safety record.

### 7. A comparison of low-risk pregnant women booked for delivery in two systems of care: shared care (consultant) and integrated general practice unit

### I. Obstetrical procedures and neonatal outcome

Klein M et al 1983 BJObs&Gyn 90: 118–122

### II. Labour and delivery management and neonatal outcome

Klein M et al 1983 BJObs&Gyn 90: 123–128

Induction, epidurals, forceps and infant intubation rates were all significantly less in the GP Unit. In the GP Unit there was less Pethidine used, less monitoring, less augmentation of labour, and the APGAR score was <6 in 17.5% of babies born in the consultant unit compared with only 1.6% in the GP unit.

### 8. Place of birth and perinatal mortality

Tew M 1985 JRCGP 35: 390–394

Analysis of published results of national surveys and specific results point to the conclusion that perinatal mortality is significantly higher in consultant units than in GP units or at home, even after allowance is made for the greater proportion of consultant bookings at high pre-delivery risk.

### 9. Five year prospective survey of risk of booking for a home birth in Essex

Shearer J M L 1985 BMJ 291: 1478–1480

With matched, low-risk groups there was no evidence of an increased risk with home confinements and there were fewer inductions, episiotomies, second degree tears, and better APGAR scores at home.

### 10. Booking for maternity care – a comparison of two systems

RCGP 1985 Occasional Paper 31

Again matched, low-risk groups. No evidence of advantage or risk in being delivered in a GP unit and greater continuity of care.

### 11. GP obstetrics: safe but endangered

Jewell D 1985 BMJ 291: 711–712

If it's safe after all, why don't more GPs do it?

### 12. General practitioner obstetrics in Bradford

Bryce F C et al 1990 BMJ 300: 725–727 and letters 1990 BMJ 300: 1139–1141

Fascinating – how to avoid cooperation between specialists and GPs, and how not to audit GP obstetrics.

### 13. Perinatal mortality rates in isolated general practitioner maternity units

Sangala V et al 1990 BMJ 301: 418–420 and letters 1990 BMJ 301: 664–667

'Higher perinatal mortality in isolated GP units' was the conclusion of the paper but once again the design, statistical methods and interpretation of the results obtained are disputed.

### 14. Community obstetric care in west Berkshire

Street P et al 1991 BMJ 302: 698–700

1989 perinatal mortality rates: community care 5.0; consultant care 8.2. 'Antenatal care of low risk pregnant women may be safely provided by their general practitioner and midwife.'

### 15. Contribution of general practitioners to hospital intrapartum care in maternity

units in England and Wales in 1988

Smith L F P, Jewell D 1991 BMJ 302: 13–16

In this survey of all the maternity units in England and Wales the authors document further the declining involvement of general practitioners in hospital obstetric care. They conclude that 'alongside' units may produce the necessary involvement of GPs in management of the unit, developing the unit's clinical policies and involvement in audit whilst retaining the unit's individual identity as well as being able to transfer to consultant care safely and swiftly.

## 16. Outcome of planned home births in an inner city practice

Ford C, Iliffe S, Franklin O 1991 BMJ 303: 1517–1519

Home births are safe when requested by multips. Primips are more likely to need transfer because of delay in labour. Close cooperation is required between GPs, midwives and the hospital obstetricians to minimise the risks of trials of labour at home. Tremendous commitment from the GPs, but the authors modestly omit this prerequisite.

## 17. Choice and change in low-risk maternity care

Campbell R, MacFarlane A, Cavenagh S 1991 BMJ Editorial 303: 1487–1488

This overview of the current evidence suggests GP obstetrics is back on the agenda, partly through the publication of evidence on safety and partly through consumer pressure.

## 18. GP trainees' views on hospital obstetric vocational training

Smith L F P 1991 BMJ 303: 1447–1452

Trainees who had done 6 months as an SHO perceived that their intrapartum competence and skills were greater than the group without the benefit of that experience. Despite this experience only two thirds felt confident about handling routine intrapartum problems e.g. resuscitating a neonate. Only one third were likely to consider using the training acquired and providing intrapartum care as GPs.

## 19. Roles, risks and responsibilities in maternity care: trainees' beliefs and the effects of practice obstetric training

Smith L F P 1992 BMJ 304: 1613–1615

More evidence that trainees see GP intrapartum obstetrics as a high risk activity. Those exposed to the provision of full obstetric care in their training practices developed a more positive attitude towards such care. However, can we or should we be expected to be at the maternity unit four times in a night and then work the next day, and will all those who cover for us out of hours be prepared to cover obstetrics?

# Work patterns in general practice

## Key questions

- Does the length of consultations in general practice matter?

- How do you feel when your surgery is running 40 minutes late?

- How do the patients feel when the surgery is running late?

- Does this matter?

- What can you do so you feel under less pressure when consulting?

- Define accessibility and availability

- What arrangements does your practice make for telephone consultations?

- Is this important?

- What are the advantages and disadvantages of personal lists?

- What would be your ideal list size? Why?

- How big a practice would be your ideal? Why?

- What sort of consultations do you enjoy least? Why?

## 1. Consultation rates among middle aged men in general practice over three years

Cook D G et al 1990 BMJ 301: 647–650

This initial survey suggests that practices need to approach a third of middle-aged men in order to offer a 3-yearly health promotion consultation.

## 2. Why consultation costs in general practice vary

Twaddle S E J et al 1990 BMJ 301: 644–645

Prescribing down by 10% = 6.8% reduction in overall costs.

Referrals to OPD down by 10% = 4.4% reduction in overall costs.

Similar decreases in diagnostic tests and radiography would produce negligible savings. Budget holders take note!

## 3. Effect of a general practitioner's consulting style on patient's satisfaction: a controlled study

Savage R, Armstrong D 1990 BMJ 301: 969–970

Simple physical illness that conforms to the biomedical model is best dealt with by a directing style of consultation. However, other problems do not benefit from this approach, particularly chronic and psychological, and a sharing type of consultation may be more appropriate. Do doctors change their consulting style according to the problems presented to them by patients? See Byrne & Long 1976.

## 4. How much personal care in four group practices?

Freeman G K, Richards S C 1990 BMJ 301: 1028–1030

Continuity of care may be fairly low in group practice, especially for children and the normally healthy. The concept of a named personal doctor may be out of step with reality in these practices and highlights the need for agreed clinical policies within groups.

## 5. Referral to hospital: can we do better?

Marrinker M et al 1988 BMJ 297: 461–464

## 6. Five years of heartsink patients in general practice

O'Dowd T 1988 BMJ 297: 528–530

A look at the outcome for the high demand chronic attender and suggestions for management strategies.

## 7. The consultation and health outcomes

Horder J, Moore G T 1990 BJGP 40: 442–443

An editorial reviewing the literature relating to the consultation behaviour finds some evidence, chiefly from North America, that there are discrete teachable parts of the consultation that have powerful beneficial effects on important measurable behavioural and physiological outcomes.

## 8. Long to short consultation ratio: a proxy measure of quality of care for general practice

Howie J et al 1991 BJGP 41: 48–54

In long consultations, independent of the 85 doctors' own styles, more psychosocial problems were tackled, more long term health problems were dealt with and more health promotion was undertaken. 10 minute appointments rule OK!

## 9. Violence in general practice: a survey of general practitioners' views

Hobbs F D R 1991 BMJ 302: 329–332

63% of responders had experienced abuse or violence in the preceding 12 months; over 90% comprised verbal threats or abuse; 66% of injuries to doctors were received during night calls. Preventative measures to consider are training in interpersonal skills and in recognising anxious and intoxicated patients, improving surgery quality and design and not keeping patients waiting for long periods to be seen.

## 10. General medical practitioners' workload survey 1989–90

Report by the Doctors' and Dentists' Review Body 1991 Department of Health

This is a very detailed report. Some extracts are:

On average, GPs work 37.01 h per week on General Medical Services and 60.49 h per week including on-call time. With other duties, the average GP's working week is 72 h.

Of this time, 16.32 h were spent doing surgeries: 8.88 h doing home visits;

5.24 h discussing cases and doing paperwork;

2.28 h on practice administration
and 1.56 h reading.

The average number of consultations per week was 163 (174 in 1985–6), but the average length of consultations increased from 7 to 9 mins over the same period. Larger lists meant more but shorter consultations.

## 11. How well do family practitioner committee and general practice records agree? Experience in a semi-rural practice

Voss S N, Thomas H F 1991 BJGP 41: 293–294

30% of addresses were incorrect, a third of the mistakes would have resulted in a letter failing to be correctly delivered. 9.4% had an incorrect date of birth and 6.6% had an incorrect name. 8% had a discrepancy involving NHS number. The majority of mistakes were in the FHSA records. This has major implications as GPs move towards electronic transfer of information and increasingly adopt an active role in contacting patients for health-screening procedures such as cervical cytology and mammography.

## 12. Factors influencing waiting times and consultation times in general practice

Heaney D J, Howie J R, Porter A M D 1991 BJGP 41: 315–319

Another paper from the Edinburgh Department of General Practice on this topic. The authors conclude that reducing waiting times is a key issue in the provision of quality services for patients and for improving the working environment of doctors.

## 13. Caring for larger lists

Marsh G N 1991 BMJ 303: 1312–1316

Introduced at a meeting many years ago as 'Britain's GP stimulator' this is another challenging article. Should this style of practice be the universal model? What are the resource and manpower implications?

## 14. Children seen frequently out of hours in one general practice

Morrison J M, Gilmour H, Sullivan F 1991 BMJ 303: 1111–1114

Not surprisingly, the socially disadvantaged were more likely to be seen out of hours. Is this demand or need?

## 15. Workload of general practitioners before and after the new contract

Hannay D, Usherwood T, Platts M 1992 BMJ 304: 615–618

A significant increase in patients seen in clinics is (surprisingly) the only measurable difference in the working weeks of Sheffield GPs.

## 16. Use made of chronic disease surveillance consultations in general practice

Beale N, Searle M, Woodman J 1992 BJGP 42: 51–53

In 43% of chronic disease consultations at least one additional item of significant clinical content was recorded. 23% of the additional items required a prescription and 7% required referral. Health promotion clinics may not be the flexible approach that patients require – particularly if delegated to practice nurses without significant additional training.

## 17. Provision of health promotion clinics in relation to population need: another example of the inverse care law?

Gillam S J 1992 BJGP 42: 54–56

Electoral wards where the standardised mortality ratio is greater than 100 or where practices were receiving deprivation payments were less likely to be offering clinics. The deprived areas had a larger number of single handed doctors.

### 18. Continuity of care in general practice: effect on patient satisfaction

Hjortdahl P, Laerum E 1992 BMJ 304: 1287–1290

In Norwegian general practice in 1987 a personal doctor-patient relationship increased the chances of the patient being satisfied with the consultation sevenfold.

### 19. Ten-minute appointments: still a challenge?

Wilson A (editorial) 15 June 1992 Update pp 1103–1106

A succinct review of the pros and cons of longer appointments. How long would you like your doctor to be able to spend with you?

### 20. Attitudes to medical care, the organisation of work, and stress among general practitioners

Howie J R et al 1992 BJGP 42: 181–185

It's that man John Howie from Edinburgh again! Doctors with a patient-centred consulting style find their work twice as stressful as those with a doctor-centred style. Longer booking intervals remove much of that stress.

### 21. Patient access to general practitioners by telephone: the doctor's view

Hallam L 1992 BJGP 42: 186–189

### 22. Evaluation of the use and usefulness of telephone consultations in one general practice

Nagle J P et al 1992 BJGP 42: 190–193

### 23. Usefulness of telephone consultations in general practice

Virji AN 1992 BJGP 42: 179–180

Two papers and an editorial on the use of the telephone in one journal! Patients find the service useful. Doctors need to find ways of meeting this demand without disrupting their existing work.

### 24. Changes resulting from increasing appointment length: practical and theoretical issues

Campbell J L, Howie J G R 1992 BJGP 42: 276–278

This paper analyses the experience of one urban practice as it changed from 7.5 to 10 minute consultations. Most objectives were achieved but, as happens so often, the practice found there were still demands on the system from having to fit in extra patients. Starting on Monday morning with sufficient appointments to meet the expected demand sounds terribly obvious but how many practices know whether they have 11 unbooked patients per 1000 registered patients at the start of the week?

### 25. General practice in Gloucestershire, Avon and Somerset: explaining variation in standards

Baker R 1992 BJGP 42: 415–418

The inverse care law again. Being a training practice, having a practice manager, younger mean age of partners, larger practice list size and a lower Jarman underprivileged area score were all associated with a wider range of services offered and a more structured and proactive approach to general practice. The author correlates this to practice development and, by implication, better care. If this is so, will current general practice changes such as GP fundholding increase or decrease the difference in services offered?

### 26. General practice partnerships: till death us do part?

Snowie N G 1992 BMJ 305: 398–400

This postal questionnaire discovered that 14% of newly appointed partners had previously been a principal in general practice. This is much higher than had previously been supposed – perhaps the traditional image of settling down into one practice for one's whole medical career is something else that is rapidly changing. The other interesting statistic was that 23% of vacancies arose because a partner was either changing career or emigrating. Didn't a health minister state recently that all was fine with general practice?

### 27. Getting to see your GP

Which? Consumers Association, Dept A103, PO Box 44, Hertford X, SG14 1SH

A challenging review of appointment and open access systems operated by six practices in one FHSA area. The results are based on interviews with 300 patients and whilst some doctors might challenge the recommendations and conclusions, there is much food for thought for those trying to match patient demand to finite resources.

## Prevention

### Key questions

- Define prevalence and incidence.

- What are Wilson's Criteria?

- Are preventative activities in general practice in accordance with them? If some are not, why have they been introduced? Why do we continue with them?

- What are the most useful prevention tasks a GP can do? Justify your choices.

- Are there risks to patients from increasing prevention activities in general practice?

- What doctor-related obstacles are there to prevention?

- How can these be overcome?

- What patient-related obstacles to prevention operate?

### 1. Using nurses for preventative activities with computer assisted follow up: a randomised controlled trial

Robson J et al 1989 BMJ 298: 433–436

Health Promotion Nurses are becoming more widely used in British general practice. The improvement obtained in blood pressure recording and in uptake of cervical cytology is impressive in a deprived area but involved tremendous effort, time and cost. Interventional screening on a large scale needs resourcing.

### 2. Mortality in relation to smoking: 20 years' observations on male British doctors

Doll R, Peto R 1976 BMJ 2: 1525–1536

A classic paper describing succinctly the evidence against tobacco.

### 3. Preventative care card for general practice

Grundy R, Dwyer D 1989 JRCGP 39: 15–16

An interesting innovation – one possible way of improving the recording of preventative data in manual records.

### 4. A handout about tetanus immunisation: influence on immunisation rate in general practice

Cates C 1990 BMJ 300: 789–790

Doctors giving out a handout are more successful in initiating a change in patient behaviour than receptionists.

### 5. A total audit of preventative procedures in 45 practices caring for 430 000 patients

Lawrence M et al 1990 BMJ 300: 1501–1503

Apart from a few shining exceptions, most practices with computers still have a large recording deficit when their preventative data is studied. Terminals on the doctor's desk, smaller partnerships and smaller doctor's list sizes were associated with better performance.

### 6. How to develop a clinical policy

Martin P / December 1984 Pulse

Many practices now use protocols for the management of diseases, usually the common chronic diseases such as diabetes, hypertension and asthma. This record is interesting because of the date. The author claims 10 years of developing practice protocols (by 1984!) and it shows. A very impressive article – a tribute to quality general practice.

### 7. Psychological costs of screening

Marteau T 1989 BMJ 299: 527

An editorial on the negative effects of screening, describing the need for monitoring the emotional and behavioural consequences as more screening programmes are set up.

### 8. Costs and benefits of inviting infrequent attenders to a 3-yearly check-up

Thompson N F 1990 BJGP 40: 16–18

Costs and benefits are often hard to establish in medicine. These rather depressing results (one mild hypertensive and three tetanus vaccinations from a list of 1448 patients requiring 28 hours of staff time and 15 hours of GP's time to organise and run the screening programme) give little encouragement to those supporting this activity. However....

### 9. Relation between use of health check ups starting in middle age and demand for inpatient care by elderly people in Japan

Tatara K et al 1991 BMJ 302: 615–618

### Health check ups for all?

Marmot M G, Haines A 1991 BMJ leader 302: 604–605

... this controversial paper from Japan shows that more check ups = less in patient care. The jury is still out and some of them are pretty sceptical, but watch this space.

### 10. Routine examination in the neonatal period

Moss G D et al 1991 BMJ 302: 878–879

An abnormality was detected on 8.8% of initial examinations. Only 0.5% of second examinations resulted in the detection of a new significant abnormality and four out of these seven were dislocated hips. A second thorough examination is therefore not necessary, though a second hip-check in the first week of life is.

### 11. Setting up consensus standards for the care of patients in general practice

Farmer A 1991 BJGP 41: 135–136

'...the development of clinical policies is likely to dominate the work of the medical profession over the next two decades.' Might be as well to make a start and read this editorial then!

### 12. Prevention in general practice: the views of doctors in the Oxford region

Coulter A, Schofield T 1991 BJGP 41: 140–143

The new contract's aims of encouraging systematic screening for risk factors and life-style advice for all patients (whether they want it or not?) were apparently not being embraced by the Oxford region's GPs, despite their considerable enthusiasm for their role in preventative care.

### 13. Prevalence and risk factors for heart disease in OXCHECK trial: implications for screening in primary care

Imperial Cancer Research Fund Oxcheck Study Group 1991 BMJ 302: 1057–1060

The purpose of the OXCHECK trial is to ascertain whether health checks by nurses have any place in the prevention of premature death from heart disease, stroke and cancer. The main indicators for cardiovascular disease present a depressing picture, maximising patient recruitment to prevention programmes remains a problem, even with intensive efforts, and the follow-up workload and cost implications are higher than previously demonstrated. Health checks are only a start – the challenge is to provide effective intervention and follow-up.

### 14. The potential and limitations of opportunistic screening: data from a

**computer simulation of a general practice screening programme**

Norman P, Fitter M 1991 BJGP 41: 188–191

The results suggest that a combination of opportunistic screening together with selected formal invitation of patient groups will be necessary to provide an adequate uptake in screening programmes. One can see from the last three papers where the arrangements for the 1993 version of health promotion have some of their origins.

## 15. Twenty-five years of case finding and audit in a socially deprived community

Tudor Hart J et al 1991 BMJ 302: 1509–1513

Organised case finding and audit resulted in fewer men who said they smoked and better care of hypertension and diabetes. The standardised mortality ratio was much lower in the under-65s than expected. This was achieved by a labour intensive approach combining accessibility, flexibility and continuity together with a planned and structured approach. Opportunistic screening was more effective than clinics, though clinics were useful for follow-up. A wonderful example to us all.

## 16. Smoking epidemiology

Fowler G 1991 The Practitioner 235: 593

## 17. Practical ways to stop smoking

Trenchard-Mabere E 1991 The Practitioner 235: 610–611

## 18. Health promotion in the general practice consultation: a minute makes a difference

Wilson A et al 1992 BMJ 304: 227–230

Recording of blood pressure, smoking, alcohol consumption, and advice about immunisation were all significantly more frequent in surgeries booked with 10 minute consultations than in the control surgeries booked at the doctor's normal rate (mean 6 minutes per consultation).

The actual length of consultations was 7.04 and 7.16 minutes in the control sessions and 8.25 in the 10 minute consultation surgeries. Why does a minute make such a difference? See also the section on 'Work Patterns'.

## 19. Three year medical checks: put medical integrity first

D'Souza M F 1 February 1992 Pulse

One of the most thought provoking articles for some time. Dr D'Souza has spent 20 years investigating the effect of screening programmes. His conclusion is that there is no evidence to substantiate the current spate of health promotion, be it 3 year checks or anything else yet reported. What evidence there is actually indicates that the effect of screening programmes is to INCREASE mortality and morbidity! It seems so important to maintain an appropriate critical attitude in this area that the source references are reproduced below:

Olsen D M, Lane R L, Procter P H 1976 A controlled trial of multiphasic screening. New England Journal of Medicine 294: 17

Lannerstad O et al 1977 Effects of a health screening on mortality and causes of death in middle-aged men. Scandinavian Journal of Social Medicine 5: 137–140

The South-East London Screening Group 1977 A controlled trial of multiphasic screening in middle age. International Journal of Epidemiology 6: 4, 357–363

Haynes B R et al 1978 Absenteeism from work after the detection and labelling of hypertensives. New England Journal of Medicine 229; 14: 741–744

D'Souza M F, Swan A V, Shannon D J 1976 A long term controlled trial of screening for hypertension in general practice. The Lancet 1228–1231 (5 June)

Hypertension Detection and Follow-up Program Co-operative Group 1979. Five year findings of the hypertensive detection and follow-up programme. Mortality by race, sex and age. JAMA 242: 2572–2577

### 20. Health promotion clinic protocols

Blackburn J Part 1 5 October 1991; Part 2 12th October 1991. Pulse

### 21. A managed approach to asthma

Henderson R 8 November 1991 Medical Monitor

Familiarity with protocols and their use is now an established part of modern British general practice. These are further examples of excellent quality.

### 22. Comparison of immunisation rates in general practice and child health clinics

Li J, Taylor B 1991 BMJ 303: 1035–1038

GPs do it better!

### 23. Primary school immunisation in Grampian: progress and the 1990 contract

Ritchie L D et al 1992 BMJ 304: 816–819

Interesting graphs on p 817 clearly demonstrate that the improvement in immunisation uptake preceded the new contract by at least 4 years! The reasons may be complex but my personal belief is that much of the improvement is down to better practice organisation and particularly the use of computers.

### 24. Facilitating prevention in primary care

Mant D 1992 BMJ 304: 652–653

Facilitators in primary care are able, by personal contact with physicians, to increase the number of preventative activities the physicians perform. The problem, as David Mant rightly points out, is that an adequate scientific basis for the activities they are promoting may be lacking. Enthusiasm, even for inappropriate activities, is always easier to facilitate than restraint – particularly when most consumers are poor choosers of appropriate medical care.

### 25. Determinants of outcome in smoking cessation

Lennox A S 1992 BJGP 42: 247–252

This is a review article which attempts to summarise what works. Methodological differences, particularly when assessing success at stopping smoking, make interpretation difficult. However, it would seem that success is in proportion to the level of input – a series of group sessions stands a greater chance of success than a chat with a GP and a leaflet. Just the chat reduces the proportion able to give up even more. Perhaps there is something to be said for health promotion clinics after all!

### 26. Lifestyle advice in general practice: rates recalled by patients

Silagy C et al 1992 BMJ 305: 871–874

More methodological difficulties dog this paper. However, the finding of extremely low rates of recollection by patients of having received lifestyle advice in general practice means there is either a lot of advice being given and then forgotten or scope for more advice to be offered.

### 27. The effect of tobacco advertising on tobacco consumption

Smee C et al 1992 Health Trends 24: 111–112

Written by economic advisers in the Department of Health, this paper concludes that tobacco advertising does have a positive effect on consumption and agrees that in four countries that have implemented a ban on tobacco advertising, the ban was followed by a fall in consumption that cannot be reasonably attributed to other factors. Can health ministers read?

### 28. Prostate cancer: to screen or not to screen?

Schroder F H 1993 BMJ Editorial 306: 407–408

Pressure is increasing from patients and doctors for the introduction of yet another screening programme without clear benefits from prospective studies.

# Alcohol

## Key questions

- How serious a problem is alcohol dependency in the community?

- How can you identify patients with an alcohol problem in general practice?

- How can you help them?

- What support services are available locally?

- What support is available for the families of patients with alcohol dependency?

- Are doctors at risk themselves from alcoholism?

- What could you do if you identified a colleague as having a 'drink problem'?

1. **ABC of alcohol**
   1988 BMJ Books 2nd edn.

2. **Alcohol – a balanced view**
   1986 RCGP report

3. **Randomised controlled trial of GP intervention in patients with excessive alcohol consumption**

   Wallace P et al 1988 BMJ 297: 663–668

Encourages and provides evidence justifying GPs and members of the PHCTs including counselling about alcohol consumption in their preventative activities.

4. **Women and alcohol**

   Dunne F 15 September 1990 Update

A review highlighting the need for the identification, and describing the possible modes of presentation, of an increasing number of female problem drinkers, together with a discussion of management.

5. **Alcohol epidemiology**

   Anderson P 1991 The Practitioner 235: 594

6. **Alcohol problems in the general hospital**

   1991 Drug and Therapeutics Bulletin 29: 69–71

7. **Alcohol and cardiovascular disease: the status of the U shaped curve**

   Marmot M, Brunner E 1991 BMJ 303: 565–568

The increased mortality amongst non-drinkers may be explained by subjects stopping drinking completely when they become ill – after the damage is done ('the sick quitter'). A public health campaign to provide cardioprotection by increased alcohol consumption will do more harm than good.

8. **Change in alcohol consumption and risk of death from all causes and from ischaemic heart disease**

   Lazarus N B et al 1991 BMJ 303: 553–556

More evidence for the significance of the 'sick-quitter' being an important influence in mortality statistics concerning alcohol.

9. **Alcoholism: a treatment plan to copy or compare**

   Cowley N 2 March 1993 MIMS Magazine

Common-sense treatment plans for these difficult problems are few and far between. This is excellent.

10. **Screening for patients at risk of alcohol related problems: the results of the York District Hospital alcohol study**

    Rowland N et al 1992 Health Trends 24: 99–102

17% of men and 3% of women were detected as having an alcohol problem in this study. With a little training in the use of screening questions it is possible to identify this often hidden factor.

# Computers

## Key questions

- What are the advantages of computers in general practice?

- What are the disadvantages of computers in general practice?

– What would you look for in a top-quality GP computer system?

– Do patients like their doctors to have a computer on their desks?

– What factors are currently limiting the progress with GP computing?

– How do practices finance their computers?

– Should they get more or less help from the FHSA/Health Board?

– How would you develop GP computing?

## 1. Computers. A guide to choosing and using

Willis A, Stewart T 1989 Practical guides for general practice. Oxford Medical Publications
133 pages including Appendix, Bibliography and Glossary of Terms.

The pace of computing in general and GP-computing in particular is hectic. General principles, however, remain unchanged. Most GPs, whether absolute beginners or computing experts, should learn important new information from this excellent little book. Hands-on experience and up-to-date information gained informally from a range of experienced computer users must, however, complement reading material.

## 2. Which computer is best for you?

A Herd and A Daniels  May 1990
Medeconomics

Those practices without a computer and those considering upgrading or changing systems could do worse than start with this article and the review of available systems therein. Once again, beware! The details degrade rapidly in accuracy with time. Get (hopefully) impartial advice from the FHSA computer facilitator (or similar title).

## 3. Computer assisted screening: effect on the patient and his consultation

Pringle M et al 1985 BMJ 290: 1709–1712

Forgive the sexist title. The initial impact of the computer in the consulting room produced a six-fold increase in the number of potentially relevant procedures. The computer was acceptable to patients and produced no increase in the length of the consultation.

## 4. Prescribing costs when computers are used to issue all prescriptions

Donald J B 1989 BMJ  299: 28–30

A personal computerised formulary reduced prescribing costs by 20–30%

## 5. The new agenda for general practice computing

Pringle M 1990 BMJ  301: 827–828

Now that basic data storage and administration are possible, future key aspects should be the computerised clinical record, communications and quality of patient care.

## 6. Large computer databases in general practice

Pringle M, Hobbs R 1991 BMJ Editorial  302: 741–742

More discussion concerning the variability in quality and quantity of data recorded by general practitioners. Only one in three practices was able to record to an adequate standard, 5% could not supply data on list size, and in one winter month 20% of practices recorded no respiratory infections.

## 7. Computerization of primary care in Wales

Goves J R et al 1991 BMJ  303: 93–94

Practices with a computer varied from 40-85% depending on FHSA. Almost half had a computer on each doctor's desk but less than 15% claimed to have full patient notes on computer. Lots of under-utilised potential – how could more sophisticated use be encouraged?

## 8. Communications – someone to talk to

Herd A June 1991 Modern Medicine pp 301–302

A discussion of the possibilities for electronic data transmission and a description of some of the pilot programmes underway. Will mainstream general practice be ready to take full advantage of the technology when it becomes widely available?

### 9. We don't have a computer

Stanley P H 1991 BMJ 303: 971–972

A challenging personal view which generated a surprisingly small amount of correspondence but which is worth reviewing.

### 10. Difficulties of analysing data

Hayes G M 1 July 1992 Update 52–59

A timely reminder. Some practices have reached the stage of having a reasonable amount of data on their computers. The problems are that even basic patient details on the practice computer may be different from other databases e.g. the FHSA or health authority records, the data on the computer may not be complete (are we sure we have entered all the diabetics into the morbidity register?) and even more insidiously the numbers of patients involved in individual practices may be so small that inappropriate analyses and conclusions result.

### 11. GP computer records – questions answered

Norwell N 1992 Journal of the Medical Defense Union No 2 pp 43–44

### Medical records on computer

Lyle P (letter)1992 Journal of the Medical Defense Union No 2 p 48

Dentists have had their regulations updated in 1992 and may now record all of their patient notes on their computer instead of on paper. No such amendment has yet been made to GPs' terms of service. A significant minority of practices have already or are actively considering 'going paperless'. Like so many aspects of general practice there is no simple answer. MRCGP

examiners are interested in whether candidates are aware of the issues.

### 12. Electronic communication between providers of primary and secondary care

Branger P J et al 1992 BMJ 305: 1068–1070

In this Dutch scheme 27 GPs were linked to two hospitals. The result was gratifyingly positive. Information was available faster and was more complete showing that electronic communication has the potential to improve quality of care delivered and reduce doctors' workload in processing the incoming data.

## Diabetes

### Key questions

– How do you detect maturity onset diabetes in your practice?

– How could you do it better?

– Who should care for diabetic patients?

– What groups of diabetics need to attend a diabetic clinic?

– How would it feel to have diabetes?

– How good are GPs at managing diabetes?

– How do you organise diabetic care in your practice?

– How good are you at doing it?

– What would make it better for you and your patients?

### 1. ABC of diabetes

Watkins P 1988 2nd Edn. BMJ Books

Comprehensive guide, essential reading.

### 2. A review of diabetes care initiatives in primary care settings

Wood J 1990 Health Trends 39–43

Of the six studies prior to 1990 that have undertaken a review of the care received by diabetics looked after in the community, only two have shown an acceptable standard of supervision and preventative care. None of the six studies was entirely satisfactory/comprehensive and their design varied. The evidence, up to this point, in favour of the wholesale discharge of stable diabetics from hospital clinics is at best extremely sparse and somewhat dated. As with other aspects of care, positive results seem to be associated with good organisation, communication, teamwork, enthusiasm and easy access to specialist advice.

### 3. How to do it – develop diabetic care in general practice

Gibbons R L, Saunders J 1988 BMJ 297: 187–189

Straightforward description of organisational matters and development of protocols.

### 4. Oral hypoglycaemics for diabetes: when and which?

18 February 1991 Drug and Therapeutics Bulletin Vol 29 No 4

### 5. Survey and audit of diabetes care in general practice in south London

Cesover D 1991 BJGP 41: 282–285

In 338 practices, 14% were running mini-clinics. Only 25% had a diabetes register. 77 doctors who audited their care showed that those who kept registers provided better care, together with those who made special arrangements for caring for diabetes. More support, particularly from dieticians, would improve the confidence and expertise of GPs caring for diabetes.

### 6. Self testing for diabetes mellitus

Davies M et al 1991 BMJ 303: 696–698

What a clever idea. Mail shot everyone aged 45–70 with a foil-wrapped dipstick and an explanatory covering letter, get them to test their own urine and pick up the undiagnosed mild maturity onset diabetics that we know are out there somewhere. It seems to work as well.

### 7. Can general practitioners screen their own patients for diabetic retinopathy?

R Finlay et al 1991 Health Trends 23: 104–5

Disappointingly, the answer is no...

### 8. General practice based diabetes surveillance: the views of patients

Murphy E et al 1992 BJGP 42: 279–283

...however, patients rate GPs' skills and accessibility higher than hospital doctors in the context of a structured community-based surveillance programme.

### 9. Systematic care of diabetic patients in one general practice: how much does it cost?

Koperski M 1992 BJGP 42: 370–372

More than the cost of an out-patient appointment in the local NHS Trust diabetic clinic. Can this be justified in terms of better attendance rates and greater patient satisfaction?

### 10. Prompting the clinical care of non-insulin dependent (type II) diabetic patients in an inner city area: one model of community care

Hurwitz B et al 1993 BMJ 306: 624–630

### 11. Influences on control in diabetes mellitus: patient, doctor, practice or delivery of care?

Pringle M et al 1993 BMJ 306: 630–634

### 12. Care of diabetic patients in hospital clinics and general practice clinics: a case study in Dudley

Parnell S J et al 1993 BJGP 43: 65–69

Equivalent care in the community, given good organisation.

### 13. How effective is systematic care of diabetic patients?
### A study in one general practice

Koperski M 1992 BJGP 42: 508–511

Systematic care, in this case concentrating diabetic care into a 'diabetic's day', improved diabetic control and record keeping. An interesting idea.

# The NHS reforms

### Key questions

– Have the NHS reforms helped patients?

– Have the NHS reforms helped GPs?

– Have the NHS reforms helped the government?

– Ideally, would you want to work in a fundholding practice? Justify your choice.

– Do deprivation payments improve the quality of general practice in the inner cities?

– Are target payments helpful? If so, to whom?

– What do patients want from their GP?

– What do patients need from their health service?

– How would you improve general practice in the inner cities?

With the exception of those who have been abroad or asleep since 1989, the fact that there has been a fundamental revision of the national health service in general and of general practice in particular, brought about by a new contract for general practitioners, should have not escaped anyone's attention. FPCs have been restructured into FHSAs and we are experiencing the effects of the other NHS reforms, principally indicative prescribing, budget-holding GPs, hospitals opting-out and general contracting in the hospital sector.

The situation is confused and evolving rapidly with significant changes and announcements almost weekly. The GP contract is still being interpreted differently from area to area so one's personal experience may not be generally applicable.

This creates certain difficulties for the MRCGP candidate trying to obtain an accurate picture of the NHS reforms. Not only is there nothing in the traditional textbooks of practice organisation but even worse – these previously unshakable foundations of wisdom and hard facts are now in part actually misleading and give incorrect information! For many candidates their only experience of general practice is under the new contract arrangements but so fundamental have been the changes since 1990 that their impact still reverberates around general practice. Like most GPs, the examiners will have struggled to a greater or lesser extent with these changes and candidates should be prepared to discuss the pros and cons of the changes in general or specific terms.

### 1. Survival guide to the contractual arrangements parts 1–5

Issued by the General Medical Services Committee of the BMA, 1989–90

### 2. Making sense of the new contract

Chisholm J (ed) 1990 Radcliffe Medical Press

These are probably the most painless way to get a reasonable overview of the current contract in that they are written in plain English. This makes the complex reforms and their effects easier to understand. In turn this means that the amendments to practice routines and organisation required can be looked at in context.

### 3. Working for patients – a journey into the unknown

1989 JRCGP editorial 39: 87–88

A broader view than that of the new contract and although written some time ago there is nothing inappropriate or out of date.

### 4. Looking for the missing billions

August 1989 Medeconomics

A persuasive overview promulgating a popular theory amongst doctors viz: many of the health service's problems could be solved if we were to spend the same proportion of our GNP as our near neighbours in Europe.

There is no substitute for reading the weekly GP newspapers (General Practitioner, Pulse and Doctor) together with the fortnightly/monthly journals concerned with finance and practice organisation (Medeconomics, Financial Pulse). If you have a local MRCGP study group it might be an idea to invite a local GP who is known to have a particular interest in practice organisation for a discussion over supper or a few beers in order to cover a lot of ground in a short time.

### 5. How much variation in referral rates among GPs is due to chance

1989 BMJ 298: pp 500

### 6. Comparison of criteria derived by government and patients for evaluating general practitioners, services

Smith C H, Armstrong D  299 BMJ  299: 494–496

The criteria derived by a group of patients scored significantly more highly than the criteria valued by the Department of Health.

### 7. How do people choose their doctor?

Salisbury C J  1989 BMJ  299: 608–610

Most people register with their nearest doctor and many did not register until they were ill. The findings suggest that competition between doctors is unlikely in itself to lead to an improvement in the quality of services provided.

### 8. Should general practitioners call patients by their first names?

McKinstry B 1990 301: 795–796

Most patients liked it and in this age of consumerism ....?

### 9. General practice: feeling fine, getting better

Roberts J 1991 BMJ 302: 97–100

Is the picture painted here over-optimistic? Only time will tell but this is an article to keep close at hand to read time and again when morale is in need of a boost!

### 10. Development of a questionnaire to assess patients' satisfaction with consultations in general practice

Baker R 1990 BJGP 40: 487–490

If we are going to have consumer surveys it makes sense to have reliable and valid questionnaires.

### 11. Second thoughts on the Jarman Index

Smith G D 1991BMJ Editorial  302: 359–360

### 12. Underprivileged areas and health care planning: implications of use of Jarman indicators of urban deprivation

Talbot R J 1991 BMJ  302: 383–386

The Jarman Index was originally designed as an indicator of general practitioner workload. Its extrapolation into a general indicator used to target resources into the apparent areas of greatest need was always likely to lead to problems, particularly when the calculations are based upon the 1981 census figures.

### 13. Training in minor surgery during preregistration surgical posts

Pringle M et al 1991 BMJ 302: 830–832

Only 14 out of 141 consultants had a curriculum for teaching house officers. Ninety offered less than 4 h teaching a week and 102 out of 139 trainees reported less than 2 h teaching a week. Confidence in carrying out minor surgery was low. The most appropriate setting for minor surgery training has underexploited educational potential.

### 14. Adequacy of general practitioners' premises for minor surgery

Zoltie N, Hoult G 1991 BMJ  302: 941–942

Most premises are suitable for minor surgery, providing proper record keeping occurs and someone checks the expiry date on the adrenalin. A number of other papers have highlighted the obvious need for all excised lesions to be submitted for histology.

### 15. General practices and the new contract

#### I – Reactions and impact

Bain J 1991 BMJ 302: 1183–1186

#### II – Future directions

Bain J BMJ 1991 302: 1247–1249

The six practices visited in December 1990 and January 1991 were still at the stage of adapting to the radical NHS reforms and learning how to restructure models of care within the new framework of general practice. Maintaining energy and morale were thought to be the most important requirements to achieve success.

### 16. General practice outpatient referrals; do good doctors refer more patients to hospital?

Reynolds G A et al 1991 BMJ 302: 1250–1252

A high referral rate does not necessarily imply a high level of inappropriate referral.

### 17. Doctors' perceptions of pressure from patients for referral

Armstrong D et al 1991 BMJ 302: 1186–1188

Pressure to refer seems to explain some of the variation in referral rates among general practitioners.

### 18. Characteristics of general practitioners who did not claim the first postgraduate education allowance

Murray T S et al 1991 BMJ 302: 1377

95% did claim (but what was the quality of the educational sessions they attended?). Of those who did not claim the allowance, there was a disproportionate number who were in small practices and who had been qualified more than 30 years. The maximum number of sessions attended by those who did not claim was two. Education may be one of the successes of the reforms in terms of numbers but what about this 5% and what about quality rather than collecting session points?

### 19. Building your own future – an agenda for general practice

1991 General Medical Services Committee, British Medical Association

### 20. The health of the nation – a summary of the government's proposals

1991 HMSO

These two discussion documents, both issued in the summer of 1991, are required reading for anyone trying to foresee the future of general practice.

### 21. Fundholding and cash limits in primary care: blight or blessing?

Rowland M 1991 BMJ 303: 171–172

The promise of nirvana versus the doomsday scenario. The real truth? 'Rapid changes are occurring in the NHS, and those doctors, fundholders or not, who are able to adapt to the changes will get the best deal for themselves and their patients.'

### 22. International crisis in health care

Fry J 15 October 1991 Update

This international comparison of the delivery of health care concludes with the stark message that the NHS is underfunded by almost 50% when compared with health care systems in other countries. With the exceptions of the USA and Sweden, there is a positive link with consumer satisfaction and increasing per capita expenditure. Is the Department of Health listening?

### 23. Travelling for earlier surgical treatment: the patient's view

Stewart M, Donaldson L J 1991 BJGP 41: 508–509

75% of patients would prefer to travel 33–55 miles rather than wait longer than 3 months for elective surgery.

### 24. Deprivation payments

Hobbs R 1993 BMJ Editorial 306: 534–585

Yet another call for a fresh look at incentive provision to encourage quality general practice in what are difficult circumstances.

### 25. Fundholding general practices – early successes but will they last?

Coulter A 1992 BMJ editorial 304: 397–398

### 26. Heartsink hotel revisited

McAvoy B R 1993 BMJ 306: 694–695

### 27. General practitioner fundholding: experience in Grampian

Wisely I C F 1993 BMJ 306: 695–697

### 28. The fundholding debate: should practices reconsider the decision not to fundhold

Keeley D 1993 BMJ 306: 697–698

### 29. NHS internal market 1991–2: 'Towards a balance sheet'

Petchey R 1993 BMJ 306: 699–701

### 30. Fundholding in the Northern region: the first year

Newton J et al 1993 BMJ 306: 375–378

The debate unfolds.

### 31. Provision of health promotion clinics in relation to population need: another example of the inverse care law?

Gillam S J 1992 BJGP 42: 54–56

Electoral wards where the standardised mortality ratio is greater than 100, or where practices were receiving deprivation payments, were less likely to be offering clinics. The deprived areas had a larger number of doctors working single-handed.

### 32. Unemployment rates: an alternative to the Jarman Index?

Campbell D A, Radford J M C, Burton P 1991 BMJ 303: 750–755

The Jarman Index correlated the worst of the five indices considered with measures of morbidity in the 59 electoral wards of the Central Nottinghamshire Health Authority. Guess which one the Department of Health still uses.

### 33. NHS reforms: the first six months – proof of progress or a statistical smoke-screen?

Radical Statistics Health Group 1992 BMJ 304: 705–709

Not yet enough evidence at this stage to say whether the reforms are improving the service to patients or not.

### 34. Your choices for the future. A survey of GP opinion

Electoral Reform Society of London 1992

### 35. A team future for general practice

Hayden J 1992 BMJ 304: 728–729

### 36. GPs' survey supports accreditation

Beecham L 1992 BMJ 304: 731–732

The General Medical Services Committee's survey of all working in British general practice produced a remarkable snapshot of the profession's attitudes at a critical time for our specialty. Briefly, GPs want less night work and (surprise, surprise) more pay. A salaried option as well or instead of the current independent contractor status will continue to be debated. Perhaps the most important response though was the small majority in favour of some form of professional accreditation for general practitioners throughout their careers. Out-of-hours care and the dilemma it presents of patient care versus GP's rest and recreation seems set to be near the top of the medico-political agenda for some time to come.

### 37. General practitioners' contract: the good, the bad and the slippery slope

Hannay D R (leader) 1992 BJGP 42: 178–179

Two years after the introduction of the new contract David Hannay provides a reflective and realistic review of some of the changes and the effects they have produced. Looking to the future he hopes, like many, for consent and self-regulation rather than coercion and legislation. We shall see.

### 38. Practice organisation before and after the new contract: a survey of general practices in Sheffield

Hannay D R et al 1992 BJGP 42: 517–520

More staff, more clinics, more computers. Better care?

# Audit

### Key questions

– What are the advantages of taking part in audit?

– What are the disadvantages of taking part in audit?

– Does audit help a practice?

– Does audit help patients?

– Where could you go to get help in starting audit?

– What would be a really interesting audit to do?

### 1. Survey of general practice audit in Leeds

Webb S J, Dowell A C, Heywood P 1991 BMJ 302: 390–392

Given the pressures general practitioners have experienced, this survey showed there was a reasonable amount of audit already being performed. However, there was evidence of

doctors needing help with time, organisation of audit and reviewing the outcome which the future coordinators of practice audit will have to take on board.

### 2. Monitoring of general practitioners' outpatient referral rates by Family Health Services Authorities: how practical?

Baker R 1990 Health Trends 22: 53–55

'Not very' is the answer to the question! One of the requirements of the new contract is that GPs should include details of their *number* of referrals to hospital, detailed by speciality, in their annual report which has to be submitted to the FHSA. Richard Baker shows that these figures will be meaningless unless related to the number of consultations. It will come as no surprise to students of the Department of Health's academic ability to discover that consultation rates are not part of the new contract annual report and the best that the FHSAs will be able to do will be to relate partnership rates of referral with partnership list sizes. In a journal published by the Department of Health, Dr Baker points out diplomatically that this will be 'relatively crude'!

### 3. Audit in general practice by a receptionist: a feasibility study

Essex B, Bate J 1991 BMJ 302: 573–576

In 4 hours a week a practice receptionist was able to assess the practice's performance with respect to immunisation uptake, follow-up of abnormal smears, screening for hypertension, recording smoking habits, diabetic care, follow-up care for psychotic illness, screening the elderly and appointment availability. Supervision required was 30 min per week in the first year and 15 min per week in the second year. We could do that in our practice, couldn't we? And wouldn't it be useful, interesting and even fun to have that sort of information?

### 4. Audit and standards in general practice

Baker R 1991 BMJ 303: 32–34

### 5. Effects of feedback of information on clinical practice: a review

Mugford M, Banfield P, O'Hanlon M 1991 BMJ 303: 398–402

Not surprisingly, the conclusion is to give feedback on performance quickly to identified decision-makers who have agreed to review their practice.

### 6. Computers in audit: servants or sirens?

Crombie I K, Davies H T O 1991 BMJ 303: 403–404

We should be careful to target data collection into areas where the information is required for analysis. This seems obvious but is frequently not the case.

### 7. Computers and medical audit

Hayes G M 15 February 1992 Update 329–334

Painless collection of data as part of all routine consultations seems to be a possible way forward with GP audit – do we have the time and energy for special projects anyway?

### 8. Medical audit in general practice

**I. Effect on doctors' clinical behaviour for common childhood conditions**

**II. Effect on health of patients with common childhood conditions**

North of England Study of Standards and Performance in General Practice

1992 BMJ 304: 1480–1488

This large scale study involved 3500 children presenting to 84 GP trainers with acute cough, acute vomiting, bedwetting, itchy rash and recurrent wheezy cough between 1984 and 1990. The standard setting and outcome assessments are remarkably complex but do show that setting clinical standards improved prescribing and follow-up by doctors and drug compliance and respiratory function in children with wheezy chests. Large scale audit would seem to be a

daunting task. This should not deter GPs from undertaking audit. Ordinary mortals can easily carry out small scale audits over a short period of time, obtain interesting results and enjoy themselves.

# Minor illness in general practice

### Key questions

– What are your indications for prescribing antibiotics for a sore throat?

– Why would you arrange to revisit a child with a temperature?

– Do you always prescribe antibiotics for otitis media?

– Should GPs prescribe paracetamol syrup or should they advise parents to buy it over the counter at the chemist?

– What would you say to the parents of a 3-year-old child with a temperature?

– Would your management change if they were flying to visit relations in New Zealand tomorrow morning?

– When would you admit a patient with gastroenteritis?

Somewhere in the MRCGP examination it is likely that the candidate will be examined on the management of what may appear to be a relatively minor and straightforward problem that is so common as to appear at times tedious. In the log diary viva in particular the examiners have the irritating habit of totally ignoring the rare 'fascinoma' that has been so carefully rehearsed, and instead ask about the child with the upper respiratory tract infection.

The good candidate will not only be prepared to offer a range of management plans for the given situation, but will also be able to select the best option for the particular circumstances presented and be able to justify the selection by reference to appropriate literature.

The BNF and 'Emergencies in General Practice' contain useful frameworks. The following papers are also highly recommended – some are considered the current definitive texts.

## 1. Treatment of sore throats

Whitfield M  15 February 1982 Update pp 589–595

## 2. Hot little children

Ayres R November 1988 Horizons pp 647–655

## 3. Randomised controlled trial of antibiotics in patients with cough and purulent sputum

Stott N C H, West R R 1976 BMJ 2: 556–559

## 4. A new look at respiratory illness in general practice

Howie J G R  1973 JRCGP 23: 895–904

## 5. Clinical judgement and antibiotic use in general practice

Howie J G R 1976 BMJ 2: 1061–1064

## 6. Family trends in psychotropic and antibiotic prescribing in general practice

Howie J G R, Bigg A R 1980 BMJ 280: 836–838

## 7. Antibiotics, sore throats and acute nephritis

Taylor J L, Howie J G R 1983 JRCGP 33: 783–786

## 8. Antibiotics, sore throats and rheumatic fever

Howie J G R, Foggo B A 1985 JRCGP 35: 223–224

## 9. Curing minor illness in general practice

Marsh G N 1977 BMJ 2: 1267–1269

## 10. Diagnosis and antibiotic treatment of acute otitis media: report from international primary care network

Froom J et al 1990 BMJ 300: 582–586

## 11. Otitis media with effusion: is medical management an option?

Burke P 1989 JRCGP 39: 377–382

## 12. Controversies in therapeutics: childhood otalgia: acute otitis media

Browning G G, Bain J 1990 BMJ 300: 1005–1007

All childhood otalgia may not be otitis media, diagnosis of otitis may be difficult, the infection may not be bacterial and antibiotics may not influence outcome. Analgesics and then review or antibiotics at presentation?

## 13. Chronic sinusitis

4 September 1989  Drug and Therapeutics Bulletin Vol 27 No 18

## 14. Acute red ear in children: controlled trial of non-antibotic treatment in general practice

Burke P et al 1991 BMJ 303: 558–562

This paper should provide the definitive answer on treating red ears with antibiotics or simple analgesia. Read it to find the answer but note that a significant flaw exists with the non-definition of exclusions and apparent arbitrary medium and long-term assessment points.

## 15. Management of feverish children at home

Kinmouth A-L  et al 1992 BMJ  305: 1134–1136

Giving paracetamol is more effective and more acceptable to parents than tepid sponging or removing clothing from hot children. However, sponging works quicker than paracetamol and adds to its effectiveness.

**16. Spontaneous resolution of severe chronic glue ear in children and the effect of adenoidectomy, tonsillectomy, and the insertion of ventilation tubes (grommets)**

Maw R, Bawden R 1993 BMJ 306: 756–760

A bit more than a 'minor problem' but an appropriate paper for this section. No definitive study has previously shown whether intervention for this problem is effective. Combined adenoidectomy and grommet insertion is better than either procedure alone. The best results were obtained in older children and where the parents did not smoke.

# Breast cancer screening

## Key questions

– What percentage of women develop breast cancer?

– Has the prognosis improved significantly in the last 40 years?

– Is breast self examination a sensible activity?

– What would you say to someone who has a breast lump which you suspect is malignant?

– How is the national breast screening programme organised?

– How would you advise a patient seeking advice as to whether a screening mammogram is worthwhile?

– What would you say to a woman recalled after an initial 'abnormal' screening mammogram?

**1. Breast cancer screening – the Forrest Report**

**1986 HMSO London**

The report recommended that all women between 50 and 64 would be offered mammography every 3 years in a national screening campaign.

**2. Mammographic screening and mortality from breast cancer; the Malmo mammographic screening trial**

Anderson I et al 1988 BMJ 297: 943–948

Concludes that women aged 55 and over had a 20% reduction in mortality from breast cancer in a screening programme. However, there was no overall reduction in mortality in the group offered screening (aged 45 years and over).

**3. The debate over mass mammography in Britain**

**The case against**

Skrabenek P 1988 BMJ 297: 971–972

**The case for**

Warren R 1988 BMJ 297: 969–970

**4. Controversy over mammography screening**

Reiddy J 1988 BMJ 297: 932–933

**5. Breast cancer screening**

Skrabenek P March 1990 Update pp 627–629

Having reviewed the results of the major trials and looked at the iatrogenic consequences and ethical considerations, the author comes out against mammography as a useful screening test. He calls for women to be counselled about the risks and benefits so that they can make a fully informed choice for themselves.

**6. Breast self examination; should we discourage it?**

Mant D 1989 JRCGP 39: 180–181

Having reviewed the trials and current treatment options, the author concludes that self examination is of unproven benefit. Nevertheless, it is still one way of detecting breast lumps and as such is appropriate to be taught to women on request.

**7. Self examination of the breast: is it beneficial? Meta analysis of studies investigating breast self examination and extent of disease in patients with breast cancer**

Hill D et al 1988 BMJ 297: 271–275

Concludes that the evidence is, with some reservations, just about in favour of encouraging women to practice breast self examination regularly.

### 8. Specificity of screening in UK trial of early detection of breast cancer

UK Trial of Early Detection of Breast Cancer group 1992 BMJ 304: 346–349

6% of 32 000 women were referred for further opinion after mammographic screening but only 1% needed biopsy. In real terms this means 1500 women unnecessarily sweating it out waiting to see if they had breast cancer or not, whilst it still remains arguable whether early detection improves morbidity and mortality.

# Child health surveillance

### Key questions

– What is the difference between developmental assessment and paediatric surveillance?

– What is the purpose of child health surveillance?

– Does it do any good?

– What is the practice programme for child health surveillance?

– What are its good and bad points?

– Could you improve it?

### 1. The Court Report 1976. Fit for the Future. HMSO

### 2. Healthier children – thinking prevention 1982 RCGP

### 3. The Hall Report 1989 Summary and comment – BMJ 2/12/89

It is interesting to see how these three reports have been received by general practitioners. The Court Report from the 1970s has never been implemented. Is this because (i) GPs were too busy organising and improving their practices

and (ii) there was no GP on the committee and its recommendations were inappropriate? Healthier Children – Thinking Prevention seemed a little more realistic but its recommendations were not enthusiastically followed except by a minority of practices who felt (sometimes very strongly) that paediatric surveillance was worthwhile. Many felt that it aspired to the ideal which was not the setting in which they worked, and that there was little evidence that a lot of effort put into the screening produced a demonstrable improvement in children's health. The Hall Report seems to have found more favour. Its aims and methods seem more realistic and achievable by average general practitioners – or is that because the new contract has changed our thinking? As the years go by the trend is to do less 'ticking of lists of tasks' and look at what elements are worthwhile. Is this because …

### 4. How good is general practice developmental screening?

Dearlove J, Kearney D 1990 BMJ 300: 1177–1180

…in Somerset screening the development of all children at predetermined ages has not been very useful.

### 5. Health surveillance of pre-school children

Colver A F, Steiner H 1986 BMJ 293: 258–260

### 6. Health surveillance of pre-school children: four years' experience

Colver A F 1990 BMJ 300: 1246–1248

Nevertheless, people are still enthusiastic and maintain that improvements in health are a direct result.

### 7. Developmental screening for preschool children: is it worthwhile?

Bain J 1989 JRCGP editorial 39: 133–134

The $64 000 question. Answer – we don't know, and another question is posed: do we really think we can make an impact against the rising tide of social problems?

### 8. Admission to the child health surveillance lists: the views of FHSA general managers and general practitioners

Evans A, Maskrey N & Nolan P 1991 BMJ 303: 229–232

The fact that national criteria are not being applied consistently is hardly conducive to finding any answers.

## Practice formularies

### Key questions

– What should be a GP's priorities when deciding what to prescribe?

– What are your criteria when deciding whether to use an unfamiliar drug?

– Do you have a practice formulary?

– Are practice formularies useful?

– How would you reduce the NHS drug bill?

– A consultant wishes one of your patients to receive a particular treatment of which you have little or no experience, but the hospital drug budget is limited and he cannot prescribe it. Do you agree to his request to prescribe it for your patient on an FP10?

### 1. Local drug formularies – are they worth the effort?

1989 Drug and Therapeutics Bulletin 27: 13–16

### 2. Introducing a drug formulary to general practice; effects on practice prescribing costs

Beardon P H G et al JRCGP 1987 37: 305–307

A reduction of 10% in costs was obtained despite modest compliance rates, no changeover to generic prescribing and no change in repeat prescribing.

### 3. Introduction and audit of a general practice formulary

Needham A et al 1988 JRCGP 38: 166–167

This antibiotic formulary produced savings over a year with no increase in consultations, home visits or hospital referrals.

### 4. Practice formularies, towards more rational prescribing

Essex B 1989 BMJ Editorial 298: 1052

### 5. How to produce a practice formulary (folder)

Waine C 1988 RCGP 14 Princes Gate, London SW7 1PU

### 6. Constructing a practice formulary

1991 Drug and Therapeutics Bulletin 29: 7: 25–26

Useful routine review article. No mention of simply picking a section in the British National Formulary and going through it at a practice meeting – a strategy which seems thorough and educationally very productive.

## Asthma

### Key questions

– On what guidelines should GPs base their asthma protocols?

– What are the trends in asthma morbidity and mortality?

– How could GPs improve the care of asthma?

– What do you say to the parents of a child who you have just diagnosed as asthmatic? How might they be feeling?

– When would you advise a patient to buy a nebuliser?

### 1. Asthma – still a challenge for general practice

Jones K 1989 JRCGP 39: 254–256

Improvements needed are (i) the identification of patients and the review of their diagnosis in the light of current criteria, (ii) a therapeutic plan being developed by the PHCT and (iii) the setting up of recall/ follow-up systems in practices.

## 2. Guide-lines for the management of asthma in adults:

**I - Chronic persistent asthma 1990 BMJ 301: 651–653**

**II - Acute severe asthma 1990 BMJ 301: 797–800**

**Leading article 1990 BMJ 301: 771–772**

Consensus statement by the British Thoracic Society, RCP, King's Fund Centre and the National Asthma Campaign. These were revised in 1993 - see later.

## 3. ABC of asthma

Rees & Price, 1988 2nd edn. BMA Books

## 4. Evaluation of peak flown symptoms only: self management plans for control of asthma in general practice

Charlton I et al 1990 BMJ 301: 1355–1359

A most impressive paper resulting from a trainee project showing that use of either plan led to a reduction in need for treatment for acute asthma and a reduction in the mean number of doctor consultations by a massive 75%.

## 5. Audit of the effect of a nurse run asthma clinic on workload and patient morbidity in a general practice

Charlton I et al 1991 BJGP 41: 227–231

Ian Charlton again, showing the reduction in morbidity following the introduction of a nurse run clinic. Doctor consultations down by 50%, fewer courses of oral steroids, acute nebulisations and days lost from school or work. Prescribing costs remained remarkably static.

## 6. An audit of inhaler technique among asthma patients of 34 general practitioners

Hilton S 1990 BJGP 40: 505–506

Overall 25% of patients studied had poor technique, and this in practices with a special interest in asthma. Some devices scored better than others but in a single audit of this type conclusions should not be drawn, other than to carefully monitor inhaler technique in asthmatics.

## 7. Prevalence of asthma in Melbourne schoolchildren: changes over 26 years

Robertson C F et al 1991 BMJ 302: 1116–1118

About 20% of children had wheezed in the last year. 46% of 7-year-olds had a history of asthma compared with 19.1% in 1964. The current prevalence is high and has increased substantially. Change in diagnostic labelling? Increased awareness in the population? Greater acceptance and availability of therapy?

## 8. Asthma care in general practice – time for revolution?

Jones K 1991 BJGP editorial 41: 224–226

Masterful review article. No more to be said.

## 9. Two year follow up of the management of chronic recurrent cough in children according to an asthma protocol

Spelman R 1991 BJGP 41: 406–409

Only one small study had previously been responsible for the modern policy of treating children with persistent cough with asthma therapy. All but two of the 106 children in this study responded to an asthma protocol, supporting active asthma treatment of 'chronic coughers'.

## 10. Management of acute asthma attacks in general practice

Jobanputra P, Ford A 1991 BJGP 41: 410–413

Patients and/or their doctors should appreciate the need for a review of their asthma management following emergency treatment for an exacerbation.

## 11. Targeting asthma care in general practice using a morbidity index

Jones K P et al 1992 BMJ 304: 1353–1356

This was a postal questionnaire to all patients on the practice morbidity register with the diagnosis of asthma. 7% of respondents who said they were no longer asthmatic and 8% who said they never had been asthmatic were found to be suffering a high degree of morbidity from asthma, and this is in a practice with a special interest in asthma! Opportunities for further education exist.

### 12. National asthma attack audit 1991–2

Neville R et al 1993 BMJ 306: 559–562

Management reported by GPs of their patients at variance with national guidelines.

### 13. Guidelines for the management of asthma: a summary

Statement by the British Thoracic Society, the British Paediatric Association, the Research Unit of the Royal College of Physicians of London, the King's Fund Centre, The National Asthma Campaign, the Royal College of General Practitioners, the General Practitioners in Asthma Group, the British Association of Emergency Medicine and the British Paediatric Respiratory Group

1993 BMJ 306: 776–782

Clearer, stepped charts. Keep copies in the consulting room and in the car.

### 14. Nebulisers in childhood asthma

15 March 1993 Drug and Therapeutics Bulletin 31; 6: 23–24

A spacer device is cheaper and often as effective. Parents need written instructions and all should be careful of over-relying on nebulised bronchodilators instead of appropriate prophylaxis.

## The health of doctors

### Key questions

– What sort of coping mechanisms would help a stressed GP?

– How do you cope with the pressures of being a doctor?
– What type of consultation makes your heart sink?
– How can you manage these consultations better?
– How will you stop yourself getting stale as a GP?
– How will you keep up to date?
– If you find yourself with health problems in the future, where could you seek help?

### 1. The health for general practitioners: a cause for concern?

Chambers R 1989 JRCGP 39: 179–181

Poor provision for the needs of GPs compared with other groups of workers.

### 2. Stress and GPs

Howie J 22 May 1989 The Practitioner p 717

Stress, and coping strategies.

### 3. Mental health, job satisfaction and job stress among practitioners

Cooper C et al 1989 BMJ 298: 366–370

Main stresses are the demands of the job, patient expectations, interference with family life, interruptions at work and home and dealing with administration. Concludes that there may be substantial benefit in providing a counselling service for GPs (and other health workers).

### 4. The doctor's health

November 1990 Symposium, The Practitioner Vol 234 pp 971–993

### 5. To burn out or rust out in general practice?

O'Dowd T C 1987 JRCGP 37: 290

### 6. Longer booking intervals in general practice: effects on doctors' stress and arousal

Wilson A et al 1991 BJGP 41: 184–187

Ten minute appointments put general practitioners under less stress when compared with the doctors' usual booking intervals of between 5 and 7.5 minutes

### 7. Self-reported health care over the past 10 years: a survey of general practitioners

Chambers R, Belcher J 1992 BJGP 42:153–156

Only 39% of GPs surveyed were registered with a doctor independent of them, but whatever the relationship personal health problems were to a great extent managed by themselves. One third of medical investigations were self-initiated, as were half of the referrals to specialists. Is there a need for an occupational health service for GPs?

### 8. Job stress, satisfaction, and mental health among general practitioners before and after introduction of new contract

Sutherland V J and Cooper C L 1992 BMJ 304: 1545–1548

Comparing 1987 with 1990, GPs experienced more stress from night calls, emergencies during surgery hours and interruption of family life by the telephone. Somantic anxiety and depression were both higher and job satisfaction had also decreased.

### 9. Psychological stresses of being a doctor

Whewell P 1 June 1992 Update pp 1003–4 (references continued on p.1071)

A review of the problems with some suggestions for coping and finding help.

### 10. Professional burnout

Kelly D 15 June 1992 Update pp 1163–1170

Clear-cut, lucid and succinct description of the symptoms, treatment and preventative measures. Terrific.

# The menopause – hormone replacement therapy

### Key questions

– What are the advantages and disadvantages of HRT?

– What would you say to a patient asking for HRT?

– Is HRT safe?

– Would you want to take HRT? Justify your answer.

– How can you advise a patient concerned about osteoporosis but not happy to take HRT?

– 'Patches are better for patients than tablets' says a pharmaceutical representative. Is she right?

### 1. Osteoporosis: prevention and treatment

9 January 1989 Drug and Therapeutics Bulletin Vol 27 No 1

An excellent review of current thoughts on prevention.

### 2. An oestrogen patch for hormone replacement therapy

27 November 1989 Drug and Therapeutics Bulletin Vol 27 No 24

### 3. Management of the menopause

Datom M E 1 July 1990 Update

Who should receive treatment, types of preparations and the risks of treatment.

### 4. HRT and the menopause

8 May 1990 Symposium, The Practitioner pp 469–493

### 5. Strategies for prevention of osteoporosis and hip fracture

Law M R, Wald N J, Meade T W 1991 BMJ 303: 453–459

This review article pulls together the current evidence from no less than 116 references! The conclusion is that exercise, stopping smoking and HRT are all successful but this protective effect diminishes within a few years of stopping treatment. Thus HRT, on current evidence would have to be continued indefinitely in order to influence morbidity and mortality in the older age groups where there is the greatest need.

### 6. Bone screening is ineffective

Effective Health Care, School of Public Health, Leeds University, 30 Hyde Terrace, Leeds LS2 9LN

This is the first of a series of bulletins produced jointly by the Universities of Leeds and York at the instigation of the NHS Management Executive. Just as the Drug and Therapeutics Bulletin offers 'best buy' recommendations, this series promises to examine the evidence on each topic and advise on areas where intervention is appropriate or (just as importantly) inappropriate.

### 7. Hormone replacement therapy and breast cancer, endometrial cancer and cardiovascular disease: risks and benefits

Goddard M K 1992 BJGP 42: 120-5

'Given the current status of epidemiological and medical knowledge about the side-effects of hormone replacement therapy, and also the limitations inherent in the design of many of the trials undertaken to date, it is impossible to give an unequivocal answer regarding the desirability of prescribing hormone replacement therapy'. But it helps to have the pros and cons of the argument adequately organised in the mind when faced with a decision to make with an individual patient.

### 8. Oestrogen therapy after hysterectomy

Seeley T 1992 BMJ 305: 811–812

What a wonderfully simple and elegant example of targeted and appropriate preventative medicine! Women who had a hysterectomy before the age of 50 were identified from their records. After 6 months 16 of the 19 eligible for HRT were still on treatment.

### 9. Postmenopausal hormone replacement therapy

Jacobs H S, Loeffler F E 1992 BMJ 305: 1403–1408

A comprehensive review article which highlights the many areas of current uncertainty concerning the risks and benefits of postmenopausal HRT.

# Complementary medicine

### Key questions

– Some patients like to consult alternative practitioners. Why do you think this is?

– A patient with low back pain requests your opinion as to whether a local osteopath would help him? On what do you base your reply?

– At a half day release session one of the trainees says 'At least complementary medicine has less side effects than a lot of the stuff we usually prescribe on an NHS prescription.' How would you reply?

– How do you feel when a patient you have been treating says she's been to see a homeopathic practitioner without a medical qualification?

– A local GP goes on a couple of weekend courses on acupuncture and then begins advertising his services. How would you respond?

– Where could you get more information about complementary medicine?

### 1. Conventional and complementary treatment for cancer

Cash J et al 1989 BMJ 298: 1200–1201

Oncology clinics should set up their own cancer support groups.

### 2. Alternative or additional medicine? A new dilemma for the doctor

Murray J et al 1988 JRCGP 38: 511–514

### 3. A model of cooperation between complementary and allopathic medicine in a primary care setting

Budd C et al 1990 BJGP 40: 376–378

A successful exercise to the benefit of doctors and patients – the way forward?

### 4. Survival of patients with cancer attending Bristol Cancer Help Centre

Bagenal F S et al 1990 Lancet 336: 606–610 and Letters 1990 336: 1185–1188

This controversial paper appeared to suggest that patients fared less well if they attended BCHC. It was later admitted that the study was flawed in that it was non-randomised and it is likely that the difference in mortality was due to increased severity of disease at entry to the study.

## Public health

### Key questions

– What is the inverse care law? Who first described it?

– What can a GP do to provide the best care for those who most need it?

– 'GPs in the inner cities should be salaried. They could then concentrate on medicine instead of running a business.' What do you think of this statement?

– How could you organise the primary health care team in your practice so that patients receive benefits to which they are entitled?

### 1. The Black Report
### Report of the working group on inequalities in health

### 1980 HMSO

Classic work on the differences in utilisation of health services and mortality related to social class. Recommendations made regarding health initiatives and allocations of resources.

### 2. The Acheson Report
### Public health in England
### 1988 HMSO

Recommendations for restructuring public health including the appointment in each health authority of a director of public health with consultant status and the publication by the authority of an annual report on public health.

### 3. Griffiths I and II
### HMSO

The swing towards care in the community and recommendations on how it should be funded and safeguarded.

### 4. ABC of child abuse

Meadow R 1989 BMA Books

### 5. Buttler-Sloss Report on the Cleveland Enquiry
### 1988 HMSO

The main findings and recommendations are conveniently summarised in the 1988 BMJ 297: 190–191

### 6. The Black Report on socioeconomic inequalities in health 10 years on

Smith G D et al 1990 BMJ 301: 373–377

### 7. Understanding benefits

Ennals S A series of 10 articles in the BMJ December 1990 – April 1991

### 8. The Children's Act 1989: Implications for the primary health care team

Sneath P October 1992 Horizons pp 456–461

### 9. Poor Britain

Delamothe T 1992 BMJ editorial 305: 262–264

A damning catalogue and summary of the relationship between ill health and poverty and unemployment. Not guaranteed to endear the BMJ to staunch Thatcherites.

**10. Health status of the temporarily homeless population and residents of North West Thames region**

Victor C R 1992 BMJ 305: 387–391

High utilisation of health resources is not surprisingly a characteristic of the temporarily homeless who are predominantly young, female, poor and with dependent children.

**11. Primary health care in London – changes since the Acheson Report**

Jarman B, Bosanquet N 1992 BMJ 305: 1130–1136

**12. Care in the capital: what needs to be done**

Metcalfe D 1992 BMJ 305: 1141–1144

**13. Secondary care beyond Tomlinson: an opportunity to be seized or squandered?**

Moss F, McNicol M 1992 BMJ 305: 1211–1214

**14. Community care in London: the prospects**

Jowell T 1992 BMJ 305: 1418–1420

**15. Public health in inner London**

Jacobson B 1992 BMJ 305: 1344–1347

**16. Improving London's health service**

Smith J 1993 BMJ editorial 306: 535–536

Providing high quality primary and secondary care in inner city areas is inevitably more difficult than in the leafy suburbs. Of the inner cities London has special problems with demography and the historical provision of services. The Tomlinson Report of 1992 is an attempt to define problems and suggest solutions. The debate seems set to continue for some time.

# Chronic fatigue syndrome

### Key questions

– What are your diagnostic criteria for the chronic fatigue syndrome?

– Do you think the problem is physical or psychological?

– How can you help patients with this problem?

– What is the likely prognosis?

– Where could you get more information about chronic fatigue syndrome for a patient?

**1. General practitioners' experience of the chronic fatigue syndrome**

Ho-Yen D O, McNamara I 1991 BJGP 41: 324–326

Each GP has two patients with this syndrome according to this study, and their care may require significant resources.

**2. Antidepressant therapy in the chronic fatigue syndrome**

Lynch S, Seth R, Montgomery S 1991 BJGP 41: 339–342

May be worth trying in those with moderately severe symptoms. This article is also a useful review of the literature.

**3. Chronic fatigue syndrome – current issues**

Wessely S November 1991 Current Medical Literature (General Practice), Royal Society of Medicine 2; 4: 99–105

A significant review of the literature with sensible and reassuring conclusions. 'I believe the best people to treat patients are neither microbiologists nor psychiatrists, but general practitioners.'

# Hypertension

## Key questions

- How do you organise screening for hypertension in your practice?

- Does screening for and treating hypertension do patients any good?

- What would you say to a patient who you feel should commence treatment for hypertension?

- What are your diagnostic criteria for hypertension?

- What are your priority groups for screening?

- What is your treatment protocol for hypertension?

- What do you include in your practice protocol for an annual check list for patients with hypertension?

## 1. Management of hypertension in twelve Oxford general practices

Stern D 1986 JRCGP 36: 549–551

Of patients being treated for hypertension:

- 50% had only a single reading before starting treatment

- 56% did not have their smoking habit recorded

- 69% had no record of weight

- 27% had pre-treatment blood pressure of 180/110 or less

- 56% were over 65 years.

## 2. Factfile 8/90 Treatment of hypertension

Published by the British Heart Foundation in association with the British Hypertension Society and the British Cardiac Society. An essential, authoritative consensus statement from an impeccable source on the diagnosis and management of hypertension on one side of A4!

Copies available from British Heart Foundation, 14 Fitzhardinge Street, London W1H 4DH

## 3. ABC of hypertension

1986 2nd edn. BMJ Books

Essential reading. Comprehensible and full of common-sense advice.

## 4. The treatment of mild hypertension

25 January 1988 Drug and Therapeutics Bulletin Vol 26 No 2

Reviews:

- Australian Therapeutic Trial in Mild Hypertension 1980 (Risk of stroke halved.)

- Oslo Study 1980 (Reduced incidence of stroke, neither coronary nor total mortality influenced. Only 795 patients.)

- Hypertension Detection and Follow-up Programme 1979 (Significant reduction in mortality from all causes in treated group.)

- Multiple Risk Factor Intervention Trial 1982 (Group receiving clinic-based intensive programme involving advice on diet and smoking, lipid screening and treatment of hypertension did no better than group receiving routine community health care despite better control of blood pressure in the special intervention group.)

- The Medical Research Council Trial 1985 (17 000 patients from general practices in Britain. Bendrofluazide v. Propranolol v. Placebo. Drug therapy halved incidence of stroke but no reduction in overall mortality or incidence of coronary events. 20% of men and 15% of women in the active treatment groups dropped out with side-effects.)

- International Prospective Primary Prevention Study 1985. (Modest reduction in coronary events in mild–moderate hypertension in male non-smokers if treated with a beta-blocker compared with group treated with a regime which did not include a beta-blocker.)

## 5. The treatment of hypertension in older patients

8 February 1988 Drug and Therapeutics Bulletin Vol. 26 No 3

Reviews:

– European Working Party on High Blood Pressure in the Elderly 1985. (Active treatment reduced cardiovascular deaths by 25%. However, overall mortality remained unchanged. Patients recruited entirely from hospital clinics – therefore pre-selected group unlikely to be representative.)

– Veterans Administration and Cooperative Study Group Trial 1970. (Only 81 patients. 55% reduction in cardiovascular morbidity.)

– Coope and Warrender 1986 BMJ. (50% reduction in stroke, no reduction in overall mortality.)

Further significant papers concerning hypertension in the elderly were published in 1991 and 1992 – see below:

## 6. Overdiagnosing hypertension

12 November 1988 BMJ leading article Vol 297 p. 1211

A fifth of patients with borderline hypertension may be treated unnecessarily.

## 7. Audit of hypertensive care

Kendrick A 15 January 1989 Update

Many patients diagnosed initially on inadequate grounds and poorly screened for causative factors. Screening for end-organ damage uncommon.

## 8. Practical aspects of blood pressure treatment

9 July 1991 Drug and Therapeutics Bulletin Vol 29 No 14

Another synopsis of current thinking on the diagnosis and management of hypertension, this time on two sides of A4.

## 9. Shep Cooperative Research Group. Prevention of stroke by antihypertensive drug treatment in older persons with isolated systolic hypertension

1991 JAMA 265: 3255–3264

Screening of 500 000 people identified 4736 persons over the age of 60 with a systolic blood pressure over 160 mmHg but a normal diastolic below 90 mmHg. These were allocated to a placebo group or a treatment group. The treatment consisted of chlorthalidone, to which atenolol was added if the target reduction of 20 mmHg was not achieved. After 5 years the average initial BP was reduced from 170 mmHg to 155mmHg in the placebo group and to 144 mmHg in the treatment group. There was a significant reduction in mortality from stroke and myocardial infarction and less mortality from all causes in the treatment group. Most British protocols advise a non-aggressive approach to the systolic blood pressure in older patients. Discuss!

## 10. Stopping treatment in patients with hypertension

Aylett M, Ketchin S 1991 BMJ 303: 345  and

### Withdrawing antihypertensive treatment

Burton R editorial 1991 BMJ  303: 324–325

Nine patients with essential hypertension, no end-organ damage, only taking one drug and with previously good control had their medication stopped and were monitored for the next 2 years. One relapsed but the others remained normotensive.

## 11. Medical Research Council trial of treatment of hypertension in older adults: principal results

MRC Working Party 1992 BMJ 304: 405–412

Hydrochlorothiazide and amiloride reduce the risk of stroke, coronary events and all cardiovascular events in older patients with hypertension. 4396 patients aged 65–74 were recruited with run-in blood pressures between 160–209 mmHg systolic and a diastolic of less than 155 mmHg. Atenolol did not show a reduction in cardiovascular events.

## 12. Management of elderly patients with substained hypertension

Beard K et al 1992 BMJ 304: 412–416

There is now convincing evidence from this review of six trials that in patients up to the age of 80 efforts should be made to reduce systolic pressure to 160 mmHg and diastolic pressure to 90 mmHg. Diuretics rather than beta-blockers are the treatment of choice but combinations may be needed in up to 50% of cases.

## 13. Detection and management of hypertension

Burton R 6 March 1992 Medical Monitor

Up-to-date masterly review article.

## 14. Management of hypertension

Kenny C March 1992 Horizons pp 125–129

This tutorial from 'the journal of vocational training' tackles management mainly in a series of problem solving exercises which are appropriate, enjoyable, enlightening and challenging.

## 15. Where are the guidelines for treating hypertension in elderly patients?

O'Malley K, O'Brien E 1992 BMJ editorial 305: 345–346

Recent studies provide strong evidence for active management of pressures greater than 160/90. Although clarification is needed to fine-tune the detailed protocols that will emerge, inaction cannot be justified in the face of a substantial body of opinion.

## 16. General practitioners' management of hypertension in elderly patients

Fotherby M D et al 1992 BMJ 305: 750–752

The findings emphasise the variable approaches adopted in advance of the above editorial review. These approaches were at the time quite justifiable, however, in the light of the variable evidence available until 1991.

## 17. Decision to treat mild hypertension after assessment by ambulatory monitoring and World Health recommendations Organisation

Chatellier G et al 1992 BMJ 305: 1062–1066

With ambulatory monitoring being promoted following the more widespread availability of non-invasive methods this study pours a large bucketful of cold water on the method. Basically the readings obtained do not correlate with the internationally accepted guidelines for assessing mild hypertension and so one or other method will select the wrong patients for treatment. Perhaps the standard guidelines will eventually require amendment given evidence from more ambulatory studies but for now it would seem to be an interesting research project rather than something on which to base sensible advice to most patients.

## 18. Blood pressure measurement by junior hospital doctors – a gap in medical education?

Feher M et al 1992 Health Trends 24: 59–61

The accurate measurement of blood pressure is fundamental to good clinical practice and patient management. One third of 80 junior hospital doctors acknowledged no formal training in how to measure blood pressure. More than one third demonstrated poor clinical technique. Check it out in ABC of Hypertension if in any doubt.

## 19. Screen detected high blood pressure under 40: a general practice population followed up for 21 years

Tudor Hart J 1993 BMJ 306: 437–440

Hypertension detected under the age of 40 is clearly dangerous. This paper makes one think about the age bands prioritised for screening in many protocols.

### 20. Management guidelines in essential hypertension: report of the Second Working Party of the British Hypertension Society

Sever P et al  1993 BMJ 306: 983–987

This working party reviews the available intervention studies, makes recommendations on thresholds for intervention, on pharmacological and non-pharmacological treatments, and provides guidelines on blood pressure measurement, essential investigations, referrals for specialist advice, follow up and stopping treatment. Could anyone ask for more?

### 21. Measurement error in the Hawksley random zero sphygmomanometer: what damage has been done and what can we learn?

Conroy R M et al 1993 BMJ 306: 1319–1322

So just when we think we've got a nice organised policy, along comes this paper to knock us sideways. Or does it? The standard measuring device apparently underestimates blood pressure so that a group with a threshold of 100 mmHg for treatment may have had actual blood pressures of 107.5 mmHg or above. This may alter the risk ratios in the selected groups but does it alter management of individual patients?

## Management of myocardial infarction

### Key questions

– What would be your immediate care of a patient with a probable myocardial infarction?

– Are there circumstances when you would not admit a patient with a myocardial infarction to hospital?

– How might a patient discharged from hospital after a myocardial infarction feel?

– What advice would you give to a patient convalescing from a myocardial infarction?

– What would you advise as secondary prevention?

### 1. A milestone for myocardial infarction

20-27 August 1988 BMJ leader Vol 297 pp 497–498

### 2. Factfile 9/88
### Thrombolysis for myocordial infarction

British Heart Foundation

Streptokinase reduces mortality by 25%; if given in association with aspirin there is a further reduction in mortality of 20%! (ISIS 2 trial)

### 3. Fibrinolytic drugs in myocardial infarction

13 June 1988 Drug and Therapeutics Bulletin Vol 26  No 12

Written before final ISIS 2 results published but a good background summary.

### 4. Home or hospital care for acute myocardial infarction? A survey of attitudes in the thrombolytic era

Pell A C H et al 1990 BJGP 40: 323–325

### 5. The management of suspected myocardial infarction by Scottish general practitioners with access to community beds

Liddell R et al 1990 BJGP  40: 318–322

### 6. Immediate primary care of a suspected heart attack

17 November 1986 Drug and Therapeutics Bulletin 24 (23): 89–91

Any general practitioner must be able to handle this situation with confidence and competence.

Patients, however, persist in presenting with atypical features about 50% of the time!

## 7. After the infarct

5 December 1987 BMJ leader 295: 1431–1432

Sound overall review of advice to give to, and management of, the post-infarction patient.

## 8. Use of secondary prophylaxis against myocardial infarction in the north of England

Eccles M, Brayshaw C 1991 BMJ 302: 91–92 and correspondence 302: 656–657

59% of patients discharged from hospital having survived a myocardial infarction were receiving suboptimal treatment. They were eligible for aspirin or beta-blockade or both but had not been prescribed the secondary prevention indicated. 'Doctors have a poor record of translating the findings of clinical trials into practice.'

However, subsequent correspondence (unchallenged by the authors) points out that there has been no prospective trial proving the benefits provided by aspirin and beta-blockade are additive. Furthermore the potential side-effects of beta-blockers include a reduction in exercise tolerance and a general feeling of lassitude – a situation one would wish to avoid when encouraging an aggressive response to exercise and a return to work.

## 9. Effects of intravenous magnesium in suspected acute myocardial infarction: overview of randomised trials

Teo K K et al 1991 BMJ 303: 1499–1503

A 55% reported reduction in mortality is dramatic enough to include this therapeutic option in any discussion of the management of acute myocardial infarction.

## 10. ISIS 3: The last word on thrombolysis?

Cobbe S M (leader) 1992 BMJ 304: 1454–1455

Aspirin and streptokinase are as good as the more expensive competitors and there is no advantage from adding heparin. The RCGP trial of anistreplase was subsequently curtailed early and now seems of reduced importance – the only advantage of anistreplase is that it may be given as a bolus injection which makes it more suitable should there be delay in admission to hospital.

## 11. The GREAT trial: Feasibility, safety and efficacy of domiciliary thrombolysis by general practitioners: Grampian region early anistreplase trial

The Great Group 1992 BMJ 305: 548–553

General practitioners responded promptly to emergency calls, were proficient in resuscitation and accurate in their clinical assessment. The time saved in this predominantly rural region by domiciliary thrombolysis HALVED the number of deaths 3 months after the infarct.

## 12. Time delays in provision of thrombolytic treatment in six district hospitals

Birkenhead J S 1992 BMJ 305: 445–448

The time from onset of symptoms could be reduced substantially by more effective use of the emergency services and faster provision of thrombolysis in accident and emergency departments. Some of these findings would superficially indicate that a GP's involvement resulted in a delay in initiating treatment. It is to the author's credit that this conclusion is not drawn, for my personal impression is that a delay in seeking help is an indication of atypical presentation or denial mechanism by the patient.

## 13. Thrombolytic treatment for elderly patients

Elder A T, Fox K A A 1992 BMJ editorial 305: 846–847

Another review calling for an active policy in cardiology. Age alone is not a contraindication to thrombolysis – indeed the benefits are greater in the older age groups.

### 14. ACE inhibitors after myocardial infarction

Vannan M A 1993 BMJ editorial 306: 531–532

Of benefit to patients with impaired left ventricular function.

# Lipids

### Key questions

– What are your priority groups for cholesterol screening?

– Should patients have cholesterol screening on demand?

– Does cholesterol play an important part in the pathogenesis of arterial disease?

– Are there problems with an increasing awareness of cholesterol as a health risk factor?

– Do you regard cholesterol testing as a high priority in your practice health promotion programme based on current evidence?

### 1. Management of hyperlipidaemia

16 November 1987 Drug and Therapeutics Bulletin (25)(23): 89–92

### 2. Who should have their cholesterol measured? What experts in the United Kingdom suggest

Leith D 1989 BMJ 298: 1615–1616

Concludes that in 1989 there is no national consensus! But...

### 3. Measuring blood cholesterol in primary care Factfile 1/91

### 4. Management of hyperlipidaemia Factfile 2/91

.... 2 years later these policy statements provide a logical framework given the current evidence. Factfiles are compiled by a wide range of doctors including general practitioners and by definition provide a consensus opinion not readily available from other sources. For address see Hypertension 1.

### 5. Adverse effects of hypolipidaemic drugs

June 1990 Adverse Drug Reaction Bulletin 142: 532–535

### 6. What should be done about asymptomatic hypercholesterolaemia?

Thompson G 1991 BMJ leader 302: 605–606

A discussion of the population-based strategy of dietary change v. the detection and treatment of people at risk.

### 7. Cost effectiveness of incremental programmes for lowering serum cholesterol concentration: is individual intervention worthwhile?

Kristiansen I S et al 1991 BMJ 302: 1119–1122

More evidence from this Norwegian paper that a population-based policy of healthy eating advice is worthwhile, whereas a targeted screening programme is not cost effective.

### 8. Does plasma cholesterol concentration predict mortality from coronary heart disease in elderly people?
### 18 year follow up in Whitehall study

Shipley M J et al 1991 BMJ 303: 89–92

Cholesterol concentration measured once was a predictor for death from coronary heart disease. Would lowering it have made any difference?

### 9. Serum cholesterol concentration and coronary heart disease in population (sic) with low cholesterol concentrations

Chen Z et al 1991 BMJ 303: 276–282

This interesting paper originates from cooperation between Richard Peto's MRC unit at Oxford and Shanghai physicians. The normal cholesterol concentration in Shanghai is 3.8–4.7 mmol/l. Even at these low levels those with the higher cholesterol suffer the most coronary heart disease. However, the mortality from liver cancer and other liver disease is the highest in those with the lowest cholesterol. Message – modify the diet but don't get lower than, say, 4.25 mmol/l.

### 10. Dietary reduction of serum cholesterol concentration: time to think again

Ramsey L E, Yeo W W, Jackson P R 1991 BMJ 303: 953–957 and correspondence 303: 1331–1333

Encouragement for the sceptics amongst us, but read the correspondence.

### 11. Total cholesterol, low density lipoprotein cholesterol and high density lipoprotein cholesterol and coronary heart disease in Scotland

Hargreaves A D et al 1991 BMJ 303: 678–681

Total cholesterol measurement is a useless measurement. Smoking, low HDL and high LDL concentrations were all associated with coronary events.

### 12. Doubts about preventing coronary heart disease

Oliver M F 1992 BMJ editorial 304: 393–394

### 13. Asymptomatic hypertriglycerideaemia – insufficient evidence to treat

Hulley S B, Avins A L 1992 BMJ editorial 304: 394–395

### 14. Should there be a moratorium on the use of cholesterol lowering drugs?

Smith G D & Pekkanen J 1992 BMJ 304: 431–434

Black Saturday 15 February 1992 for the advocates of lowering cholesterol as a means of significantly reducing cardiovascular disease. However, there is still a vigorous debate with an alternative view:

### 15. Preventative medicine in primary care: management of hyperlipidaemia

Lewis B 1992 BJGP Editorial 42: 47–50

### 16. Relation between coronary risk and coronary mortality in women of the Renfrew and Paisley survey – comparison with men

Isles C G et al 1992 Lancet 339: 702–706

Women had higher cholesterol levels, similar diastolic pressures and smoked less. Fatal coronary events were almost twice as likely in men and the absolute risk of women with cholesterol levels of 7.2 mmol/l was less than that of men with levels of below 5 mmol/l. 'The definitive guide-lines for the treatment of hypercholesterolaemia in women must await the result of further clinical trials.' In the meantime it would seem appropriate to be very cautious indeed about the prescribing of lipid lowering drugs to women and to reassure female patients with levels up to at least 7.2 mmol/l.

### 17. Low serum cholesterol concentration and short term mortality from injuries in men and women

Lindberg G et al 1992 BMJ 305: 277–279

Confirmation of previous studies showing a cholesterol concentration well below average is associated with an excess of violent death, principally from suicide.

### 18. Motivational effect of cholesterol measurement in general practice health checks

Robertson I et al 1992 BJGP 42: 469–472

Minimal effect demonstrated.

# Cardiology

### Key questions

– A patient attends your surgery with increasing angina. How do you assess him? What would indicate the need for referral?

– Does exercise prevent heart disease?

– A dentist rings up for advice about a patient with an aortic valve replacement who needs three teeth extracting. What would you reply?

– Outline the possible management of a patient with lone atrial fibrillation. When should ACE inhibitors be prescribed?

## 1. The management of unstable angina

5 February 1990 Drug and Therapeutics Bulletin 28 (3): 9–11

Admit to hospital for aspirin, nitrates and beta-blocker. If necessary add calcium antagonist. Refractory symptoms should then be treated with IV nitrate and consideration given to the need for urgent angiography, ? angioplasty/by-pass surgery.

## 2. Exercise in leisure time: coronary attack and death rates

Morris et al 1990 Br Heart Journal 63: 325–334

Confirms other studies in showing that vigorous, aerobic exercise has a protective effect, reducing myocardial infarction rate to less than half of other men. Less vigorous exercise also confers some benefit. However, the benefit only accrues to those whose exercise is habitual and continuing.

## 3. Coronary artery by-pass grafting for the reduction of mortality: an analysis of the trials

3 November 1984 BMJ 289: 1166–1170

Patients who can climb a flight of stairs without developing angina can safely have their angina managed medically; there is no evidence that surgery will prolong their lives. Unfortunately all three trials had design flaws.

## 4. Prophylaxis for endocarditis

15 July 1985 Drug and Theraputics Bulletin 23 (14): 53–56

Antibiotics are given because it seems a reasonable thing to do rather than on evidence of effi-cacy from clinical trials. The treatment recommendations have been superseded:

## 5. Antibiotic prophylaxis of endocarditis: new recommendations

12 November 1990 Drug and Therapeutics Bulletin 28 (23): 90–91

## 6. Risk assessment in the prevention of coronary heart disease: a policy statement

Coronary Prevention Group 1990 BJGP 40: 467–469

This is a tremendously useful summary of the current thoughts regarding useful preventative practice in this field. Julian Tudor Hart from Glyncorrwg, the late Maurice Stone from the RCGP Research Unit at Leigh and Robert Cunningham from North Yorkshire are amongst those who have shown that it is possible to make tremendous inroads into cardiovascular mortality at the level of a practice population using a combined attack on smoking, obesity, lipids and lifestyle. There are more than 30 000 deaths under the age of 64 each year from ischaemic heart disease and if general practice is to make a significant contribution to prevention in terms of numbers of lives saved this is the place to start.

## 7. Risk factors for stroke in middle aged British men

Shaper A G et al 1991 BMJ 302: 1111–1115

Nice to have confirmation from this study based in British general practice that the major risk factors are systolic blood pressure, cigarette smoking, heavy alcohol intake and left ventricular hypertrophy on the ECG in patients with known ischaemic heart disease.

## 8. Alcohol consumption and risk of coronary heart disease

Jackson R et al 1991 BMJ 303: 211–216

Light and moderate alcohol consumption really does seem to have a cardioprotective effect. Thank goodness for that.

## 9. An action plan for preventing coronary heart disease in primary care

Working Group of the Coronary Prevention Group and the British Heart Foundation 1991 BMJ 303: 748–750

## The Dundee coronary risk-disk for management of change in risk factors

Tunstall-Pedoe H 1991 BMJ 303: 744–747

Smoking, blood pressure and cholesterol readings are combined to produce a risk score for coronary disease modified for age and sex.

## 10. Alcohol consumption and its relation to cardiovasular risk factors in British women

Razay G et al 1992 BMJ 304: 80–83

Moderate alcohol consumption (1–20 g/day) is associated with lower levels of cardiovascular risk factors in women.

## 11. Management of atrial fibrillation

Pritchett E L C 1992 New England Journal of Medicine 326: 1264–1271

The author reviews three trials:

(i)   The Copenhagen Atrial Fibrillation, Aspirin, Anticoagulation Study.

Five patients in the warfarin group suffered embolic complications, compared with 20 in the aspirin group (75 mg daily) and 21 in the placebo group. Twenty-one patients had bleeding problems with warfarin, compared with only 2 in the aspirin group and none in the placebo group.

(ii)  The Boston Area Anticoagulation Trial for Atrial Fibrillation.

Warfarin treatment was associated with a stroke incidence of 0.4% a year compared with 3.0% a year in the control group.

(iii) The Stroke Prevention in Atrial Fibrillation Study.

This is the largest study and is still in progress. The annual rate of ischaemic stroke and systemic emboli is 3.6% in the aspirin group (325 mg daily), 2.3% in the warfarin group and 6.3% in the placebo group. The incidence of bleeding problems is the same in all three groups.

He concludes that anticoagulation with warfarin should now be advised in patients with atrial fibrillation unless they have a contraindication such as peptic ulceration, liver disease or frequent falls. Exceptions would be patients under the age of 60 with no other risk factors (particularly hypertension) and no other evidence of heart disease – these patients have a low incidence of embolic complications without any intervention.

## 12. Driving and the heart

Factfile 6/92 British Heart Foundation

One side of A4 for quick revision and reference.

## 13. ACE inhibitors – a cornerstone in the treatment of heart failure

Braunwald E et al 1991 New England Journal of Medicine 325: 351–353

## 14. A comparison of Enalapril with hydralazine-isosorbide dinitrate in the treatment of chronic congestive heart failure

Cohn J N et al 1991 New England Journal of Medicine 325: 303–310

## 15. Effect of Enalapril on survival in patients with reduced left ventricular ejection fractions and congestive heart failure

The SOLVD Investigators 1991 New England Journal of Medicine 325: 293–302

Following the publication of these studies ACE inhibitors deserve to be used widely and early in congestive cardiac failure. They help patients haemodynamically and clinically and improve survival.

## 16. Managing heart failure – home or hospital?

Drug and Therapeutics Bulletin 1992 Vol 30 No 16

Rather an odd title for acute heart failure clearly requires hospital admission in most circumstances whereas the non-acute presentation is almost always treatable at home. That apart, an eminently sensible review, again making a case for more widespread use of ACE inhibitors.

### 17. Carotid endarterectomy: recommendations for management of transient ischaemic attack and ischaemic stroke

Brown M M et al 1992 BMJ 305: 1071–1074

Evidence for an aggressive approach to another aspect of vascular disease. Active investigation of patients is required to identify those patients with stenoses greater than 70% who definitely benefit from expert surgery. Patients with a 30–70% stenosis are in the 'not proven' category for surgery and should if possible be entered into the ongoing trials. Medical treatment should be offered to those with a stenosis of less than 30%.

### 18. Cost effectiveness of primary stroke prevention in atrial fibrillation: Swedish national perspective

Gustafsson C et al 1992 BMJ 305: 1457–1460

### 19. Atrial fibrillation and stroke: prevalence in different types of stroke and influence on early and long term prognosis (Oxfordshire Community Stroke Project)

Sandercock P et al 1992 BMJ 305: 1460–1465

### 20. Antithrombotic treatment and atrial fibrillation

Lowe G D O 1992 BMJ Editorial 305: 1445–1446

More evidence in favour of Warfarin as a primary stroke preventer in patients with atrial fibrillation. The Oxford study indicated that the presence of atrial fibrillation in patients who had a stroke was not an additional risk factor for further vascular events – the risk is high after a stroke whatever other factors are present.

### 21. Low systolic blood pressure and self perceived well-being in middle aged men

Rosengren A et al 1993 BMJ 306: 243–246

Some studies have shown an association between low blood pressure and a variety of non-specific symptoms. This paper confirms this but the explanation is uncertain. In Germany there are many drugs marketed and prescribed for low blood pressure – cultural influences in medicine in the first world as well as the third.

# Cervical cytology

### Key questions

– Describe the recent mortality rate pattern for cancer of the cervix.

– What do you think would lead to a significant improvement in the morbidity and mortality from cancer of the cervix?

– How do you organise call and recall of cervical cytology in your practice?

– At what intervals do you offer screening? Is this appropriate on current evidence?

– Are there some circumstances when confidential care may be compromised? How do you get round these problems?

– How do you inform patients of their normal results? Could this system be improved?

– How do you inform patients of an abnormal result?

– How do you think a patient feels when her smear is reported as abnormal?

### 1. Making cervical cytology work

24 June 1989 BMJ 298: 1662–1664

Better management of the system is essential.

### 2. Cervical screening in general practice: a new scenario

Chomet J, Chomet J 1990 BMJ 300: 1504–1506 and the subsequent letters  301: 236–238

There is obviously still no agreement on the timing of the first smear, how frequent subsequent smears should be taken, how to manage the mildly abnormal smear and...

## 3. Cervical cancer screening

Skrabanek 15 April 1990 Update pp: 868–872

... even whether there is sufficient evidence that screening programmes have made a significant contribution to the decline in deaths from cervical cancer.

## 4. Prospective randomised controlled trial of methods of call and recall for cervical cytology screening

Pierce M et al. 1989 BMJ 299: 160–162

Tagging GPs' records and sending patients' records were both equally effective in doubling the numbers who had a smear test.

## 5. Evaluation of a call for cervical cytology screening in women aged 50–60

Robertson A J et al 1989 BMJ 299: 163–166

Targeting invitations to non-responders it was possible to increase the percentage of women screened from 58 to 69. A further 15% of women were identified who had a valid reason for exclusion from the programme.

## 6. Investigation of non-responders at a cervical cancer screening clinic in Manchester

Nathoo V, 1988 BMJ 296: 1041–1042

Practice uptake of an FPC call and recall system was only 14%. A sample of non-responders was investigated. More than half the non-attendance was directly attributable to administrative errors which resulted in appointments being sent to wrong addresses or to inappropriate people - 8% had a hysterectomy and 20% a recent smear.

## 7. Evaluation of the cervical cytology screening programme in an inner city health district

Beardow R et al 1989 BMJ 299: 98–100

69% of invitation letters sent out by an FPC in London were either inaccurate or inappropriate. Almost half the recorded addresses were incorrect and 20% of the women were not eligible for a test.

## 8. How district health authorities organise cervical screening

Elkind A et al 1990 BMJ 301: 915–918

Only just over half of health districts had a system which called women in the 20–65 years target age range. Only 70% expected to make the target date of 13 March 1993 for completing the call. Considerable variance was evident among the schemes with regard to population coverage, quality of testing and follow up of abnormal results.

## 9. Can health education increase uptake of cervical smear testing among Asian women?

McAvoy B R, Raza R 1991 BMJ 302: 833–836

Answer: Yes. Personal visits were the most effective; some evidence that home-viewed videos may be particularly effective in reaching Urdu speaking Pakistani Moslems. Postal leaflets were a waste of effort.

## 10. Cervical screening in Perth and Kinross since introduction of the new contract

Reid G S et al 1991 BMJ 303: 447–450

The mean percentage of women screened increased from 78% in July 1989 to 85% in October 1990, 6 months after the introduction of the new contract. Once again the single most important factor leading to this good performance is an adequate and accurate population database.

## 11. Nuns, virgins and spinsters: Rigioni-Stern and cervical cancer revisited

Griffiths M 1991 Br JOG 98: 797–802

Briefly, this fascinating paper reviews the literature which has led to the oft-quoted suggestion that cervical cancer is rare amongst nuns. The conclusion is that the evidence does not substantiate this statement and screening should be offered to groups of non-sexually active women. There is a danger of doctors and patients being falsely reassured and if suspicious symptoms occur expert examination under anaesthesia should be advised, as it would be for other groups.

## 12. Audit of practice based cervical smear programme: completion of the cycle

Creighton P A, Evans A M 1992 BMJ 304: 963–967

Evidence that practice based cervical screening programmes can be highly effective, one of the main requirements being a well-organised primary health care team. But this is a stable population in Northumberland – general practice in the inner cities is a different ball game with a shifting population and sometimes poorer organisation and support.

## 13. Abnormal cervical smear test result : old dilemmas and new directions

Wilkinson C 1992 BJGP 42: 336–339

A review that is hard to fault.

## 14. Predicting mortality from cervical cancer after negative smear test results

van Oortmarssen G J et al 1992 BMJ 305: 449–451

The authors advocate screening intervals longer than 3 years but there are plenty of others offering the contrary view.

## 15. Rationale for stopping cervical screening in women over 50

van Wijngaarden W J, Duncan I D 1993 BMJ 306: 967–971

The debate on who to screen and how often continues without consensus emerging. These authors suggest that women over 50 with a history of several negative smears at 3 year intervals can be safely discharged from further screening.

# Miscellany

This section contains details of papers and articles thought to be useful, stimulating or entertaining (preferably all three) which do not fit into one of the defined topic headings.

## 1. The gatekeeper and the wizard: a fairy tale

Mathers N, Hodgkin P 1989 BMJ 298:172–174

## 2. The gatekeeper and the wizard revisited

Mathers N, Usherwood T 1992 BMJ 304: 969–971

Perhaps these short pieces could be included in the 'NHS Reforms' section but the reader must make up their own mind. Witty and well written – an excellent relaxation from the hard grind of examination preparation.

## 3. Use of thermometers in general practice

Clarke S 1992 BMJ 304: 961–963

Your trainee project can be worth a wider audience than the local Syntex competition!

## 4. Storage of vaccines in the community: weak link in the cold chain?

Thakker Y, Woods S 1992 BMJ 304: 756–758

These last two papers are examples of how important it is to look at simple everyday activities with a critical eye.

## 5. How much do doctors know about the notification of infectious diseases?

Voss S 1992 BMJ 304: 755

The examiners' attention has been drawn to a widespread lack of basic knowledge amongst GPs and junior hospital doctors. What would you do if you were an examiner?!

### 6. Relationship between the working styles of general practitioners and the health status of their patients

Huygen F J A et al 1992 BJGP 42: 141–144

For many years RCGP-inspired GPs have been trying to move from the medical school model of practising medicine of treating diseases in a doctor-centred way towards a patient-centred approach with agreed aims between doctor and patient. This has often been accompanied by attempts at a low referring, low prescribing approach with appropriate, but not superfluous investigations. It is difficult to assess the outcome of this change in medical models accurately. Doctor and patient satisfaction are usually found to be higher but this does not imply better health as a result of the changed approach. This study from Holland involved 1500 women aged between 50 and 65 years selected from the lists of 75 GPs who had their style of medical practice previously analysed. The patients of GPs with the 'integrated style' felt more healthy, had more realistic expectations about the possibilities of professional help for common ailments, had fewer symptoms and tended to visit their doctor less frequently.

### 7. Edinburgh primary care depression study: treatment outcome, patient satisfaction and cost after 16 weeks

Scott A I F, Freeman C P L 1992 BMJ 304: 883–887

The RCGP has had a special interest in the management of depression in recent times (you have been warned). This study randomised patients with the criteria for a major depressive episode without psychosis to receive either amitriptyline from a psychiatrist, cognitive behaviour therapy from a clinical psychologist, counselling and case work from a social worker or routine care from a general practitioner. At 16 weeks there were only small advantages in the specialist treatment groups but specialist treatment involved four times as many contacts and cost twice as much as routine GP care. Marked improvement occurred in all groups. This is encouraging for GPs with low referral rates of patients with depression if long-term outcome and relapse rates are also similar.

### 8. Communication between general practitioners and consultants: what should their letters contain?

Newton J, Eccles M, Hutchinson A 1992 BMJ 304: 821–824

There have been many studies over the years into GP-consultant and consultant-GP communication. As a result of this project the authors state 'A high degree of consensus exists between clinicians...they have unambiguously endorsed a standard of communication they can aspire to.' Doctors agreeing with each other – whatever next!

### 9. Meningococcal infections: reducing the case fatality rate by giving penicillin before admission to hospital

Strang J R, Pugh E J 1992 BMJ 305: 141–143

### 10. Early treatment with parenteral penicillin in meningococcal disease

Cartwright K et al 1992 BMJ 305: 143–147

### 11. Reducing mortality from meningococcal disease

Snaith P 1992 BMJ editorial 305: 133–134

Parenteral penicillin administration as early as possible produces a significant reduction in mortality from meningococcal disease. Apparently no study has satisfactorily shown this previously and a survey in 1988 showed less than half of GPs carried injectable penicillin in their bags.

### 12. Comparison of the use of four desktop analysers in six urban general practices

Hobbs F D R et al 1992 BJGP 42: 317–321

### 13. Desktop laboratory technology for general practice

Freeman G K 1992 BJGP editorial 42: 311–312

An example of interesting technology that is probably not that useful or appropriate unless large numbers of tests are being performed on a daily basis. If your senior partner was interested in the practice buying one could you discuss the pros and cons intelligently and knowledgeably?

### 14. Pre-recorded answerphone messages: influence on patients' feelings and behaviour in out of hours requests for visits

Bennett I J 1992 BJGP 42: 373–376

Problems with the methods employed in this study leave slight doubts about the validity of the conclusions. Nevertheless a sufficiently interesting paper to merit a mention in dispatches. Patients preferred and responded most appropriately to a message recorded by a doctor in a neutral (rather than strict) tone giving details of the next surgery and what to do in an emergency.

### 15. Reaccrediting general practice

Gray D P 1992 BMJ editorial  305: 488–489

The first stirrings of a controversy that may run and run. GPs in the GMSC survey 'Your Choices For The Future' seemed to agree that basic medical qualification and the satisfactory completion of vocational training was insufficient in itself for the next 30 years as a general practitioner. The prospect, therefore, is of some form of reaccreditation procedure performed at intervals throughout the career of all general practitioners in order to ensure patients' interests are protected.  A minefield to be entered only by the brave or the foolhardy given present reports of the morale of many GPs.

### 16. Racial discrimination against doctors from ethnic minorities

Esmail A, Everington S 1993 BMJ  306: 691–692

Such discrimination is quite disgraceful. The authors are to be congratulated. They are also probably the only writers in the BMJ's history to have their survey interrupted because they were arrested by the police for making fraudulent job applications.

### 17. Low back pain

Frank A 1993 BMJ 306: 901–909

A straightforward but very useful review of a condition commonly presenting in the surgery.

### 18. Immunisation against influenza among people aged over 65 living at home in Leicestershire during winter 1991–2

Nicholson K G 1993 BMJ 306: 974–976

This paper highlights yet another aspect of the inverse care law that one suspects operates in a lot of practices. Influenza vaccine is safe and effective but requires targeting at patients with medical indications. If this does not happen then the result may be that those most in need miss out and the active, fit and motivated who ask will be the ones vaccinated instead.

# 7

# The Orals

After the written papers have been marked, the crude scores obtained are adjusted so that the marks on each paper each have a mean of around 50% and a standard deviation of approximately 10%. This is done to ensure that equal weight is given to the marks obtained in each of the three papers. Each candidate's adjusted scores are then totalled.

In recent years the pass rate for the examination as a whole has remained steady at 72–75%. The examiners do not invite the bottom 20% of candidates in the written papers to attend for the oral examinations since experience shows that those candidates have an impossible task – however well they perform in the orals it is just not possible for them to obtain enough marks to reach the eventual pass level. Equally, simple arithmetic shows that candidates a few per cent above the mean in the written papers and apparently safe can have two bad vivas and contrive to eventually fail.

The message for candidates who are invited to the orals is one of cautious hope. Their chances of passing the examination as a whole are much improved but on a purely mathematical basis the oral marks can be crucial. Knowledge of the viva format, information about the likely content, an understanding of the marking schedule and diligent preparation are still vital.

## Format

The orals are held a few weeks after the written papers in Edinburgh and London. The established format is that in Edinburgh the RCGP uses one of the other Royal Colleges as a base, whilst in London the college building at 14 Princes Gate is the obvious choice despite limited space. The majority of candidates request London as their venue so the examination panel spends 2 or 3 days in Scotland followed by a week or 10 days in London.

There are two vivas each lasting almost 30 minutes with only a short break in between. Each viva is conducted by two examiners both of whom will pose questions. There may be a third examiner present or a video camera to record the viva. Their presence is, if anything, a factor in favour of the candidate since their purpose is

131

to observe the performance of the examiners. Most candidates are pleasantly surprised at the approach from the examiners which is to try to draw out the best from the candidates. The presence of a human or electronic invigilator should act as a reminder to those on the right side of the examination table to be on their best behaviour, since eccentricities captured on videotape may be presented to the rest of their peers at the examiners meeting the next morning!

The first viva is based on the Practice Experience Questionnaire, formerly called the log diary. This consists of a structured description of the candidate's practice and a list of patients from surgeries, visits and out-of-hours calls. The second viva is a problem solving viva – the problems this time are presented by the examiners as the basis for discussion.

# Content

In the first viva the skeleton provided is used only as a skeleton. You will not be asked to describe in great detail the layout of the practice's main surgery or the minutiae of the history of patient 14 with systemic lupus erythematosis. Indeed if you spend time on lengthy descriptive passages you will be interrupted by the examiners and required to produce information which is markable. The following are examples of the type of questions which might be posed:

— 'I see that patient 3 is a boy aged six with chickenpox. Having made the diagnosis, what areas would you want to cover in the rest of that consultation?'
— 'I see that patient 3 in your surgery has chickenpox. Do your receptionists have any special advice from the practice when faced with a request for help from the parent of a child with a rash?'

Sometimes a blank canvas is offered for you to paint:

— 'Patient 3 with chickenpox. Tell me about chickenpox.'

With regard to practice equipment:

— 'I see you have a peak flow meter. Where does that fit in the management of asthma?'

— 'I see you have an ECG machine. If you are called at 1 a.m. to a 60-year-old man with chest pain is it worth making a 10 minute detour to collect the ECG from the surgery?'
— 'You have a defibrillator in the practice. What are the arguments for and against having a defibrillator?'
— 'Like many practices nowadays you have a computer. If you were about to take delivery of the practice's first computer, what preparations would you need to make?'

The practice staff:

— 'I see you have a practice manager. What skills do practice managers need?'
— 'With regard to practice nurses, what is your legal situation as a general practitioner if your practice nurse gives a patient incorrect advice or treatment?'
— 'What would you do if you, as a general practitioner, heard one of your receptionists tell a neighbour that a mutual acquaintance had just been discharged from hospital after a termination of pregnancy?'

There have been recent changes to the log diary which reflect the changing face of general practice in the last few years. The amendments relate to:

– premises
– computers
– budget-holding
– out-of-hours arrangements
– child health surveillance
– audit
– minor surgery
– special features of the practice
– health promotion clinics
– suggestions for practice changes.

The questions posed in the problem solving viva will be similarly phrased. In both vivas the examiners will spend time on the high priority areas already described in the section 'Aims and Objectives'. They also have a sheet highlighting the seven areas of competence and over the course of the vivas the two pairs of examiners will try to cover each of the seven areas with at least one series of questions. Most areas may be covered on several occasions.

Candidates preparing for the examination will be fascinated with the marking schedule for the oral examinations. It is difficult and probably unhelpful to try to extrapolate from the tables' broad categories to marks in per cent. It is, however, quite clear that a candidate who is unable or forgets to justify approaches selected by reference to the literature of general practice can at best only be awarded 'Bare Pass'. With good marks in the orals being a requirement even of candidates who have scored a little higher than the mean in the written papers, the implication is obvious – READ THE LITERATURE AND QUOTE IT AT EVERY OPPORTUNITY.

## Technique

Some practical points first of all:

### 1. Getting there

Generally speaking, it is wiser to rely upon public transport than one's own. If the train or bus breaks down there is usually an alternative method of transport available which will still get you to the examination centre in time, providing you are prudent and leave plenty of contingency time in your travel plans. If you are in your own car and are delayed by accident, mechanical failure or traffic jams it is much more difficult to extricate yourself with the minimum expenditure of adrenalin. Parking is impossible in London for visitors without influence or friends in high places. Edinburgh is not much better.

Travelling the previous evening and staying overnight near the examination centre may be worth the effort and expense and is certainly worth considering. Most people travel to Princes Gate on the underground. It is a good 10 minutes walk uphill from South Kensington station to the College – don't be caught out and have to rush the last few hundred yards in a panic since this is unlikely to improve your performance.

### 2. Not getting there

If, despite meticulous and sensible planning, you still find yourself in a situation where you think it highly likely or certain that you will be late for your allotted time, telephone the examination centre as soon as possible. It goes without saying that having the telephone number to hand in case of this eventuality would be sensible planning. This may all seem an unlikely scenario but having known a candidate fail by 1% following a dramatic last minute dash to the viva, followed by an even more dramatically poor viva – be warned. It happens to someone every year.

Some intercity trains have public telephones on the train itself. Failing that, a walk up and down may discover a fellow passenger with a cellphone. There may even be a cooperative guard who may be able to get your message relayed for you. The examination administrators are always polite, courteous and as helpful as possible. There are contingency times later in the day for just this sort of eventuality and all may not be lost given a bit of quick thinking and communicating your difficulties as early as possible.

### 3. Being there

Arrive in plenty of time, but if you get very nervous waiting it might be prudent to get to the vicinity of the examination and then kill time elsewhere, entering the building itself with perhaps 15 minutes to get your bearings. A waiting area is set aside and you may be offered a cup of coffee. Before accepting, consider the effect this might have on your bladder, gastrointestinal tract and heart rate.

Be prepared for a civilised approach from the College staff and the examiners. This is unexpected to those experienced in British undergraduate and postgraduate medical examinations; do not allow a false sense of security to undermine your determination to give of your best – they are nice to everybody!

In the vivas:

## Body language and non-verbal clues

Dress is always a controversial area. Having tried to steer clear of the issue for a time in seminars and then almost always getting a question on the subject from the audience, it seems essential to give the majority opinion as guidance, though some would disagree.

Without wishing to seem patronising, this is a serious professional examination. Most general practices are still very conservative in their approaches to dress. This may not work to their advantage but is nevertheless the case at present. The examiners are likely to come from established practices where innovation may be medically acceptable but what do we know about their dress habits? Jeans and an old sweatshirt may work well for your consulting style and the patients may respond positively to the informality. However, this is not the occasion for informality.

The minimum requirements are to look reasonably smart and clean. Something comfortable and presentable may help one feel a little more at ease. Designer suits may be slightly over the top for most candidates. This is about average general practice and not a power breakfast in a city merchant bank. Full regimental dress uniform of the Household Cavalry is certainly not required! On the other hand trainers, a pair of cords and an open neck shirt may be taking a relaxed approach to postgraduate examinations a little too literally.

One final thought is that in London in the summer it can be hot and humid. In the confined space at Princes Gate a good anti-perspirant/deodorant is worth its weight in gold and the option of lightweight but still smart clothes would be worthwhile. The examiners are unlikely to appreciate an aroma of last night's garlic and/or alcohol. If it is warm the examiners will have discarded jackets and will invite you to make yourself comfortable and do the same.

Non-verbal clues can make quite a difference to the impression the examiners have of a candidate. Practice sitting up straight in the chair rather than slumping. Look the examiners in the eye at least some of the time, try to look cheerful and keen to impress. Smile and be confident, even if you feel exactly the opposite and require a large dose of IM Stemetil! Don't fidget, do sit on your hands discreetly if they tremble a lot and don't wave them about too much – you might just send something important flying across the room.

Practise these viva skills with colleagues. It should be possible to work with others locally who are also sitting the examination. If you can borrow a camcorder, record a mock viva and play it back, either in private or better still in a group for discussion. Use the same rules that are used when viewing consultations with a few amendments:

| | |
|---|---|
| 1. Victim. What I did well | – appearance, non-verbal clues and presentation |
| | – viva content |
| What I could do better | – appearance, non-verbal clues and presentation |
| | – viva content |
| 2. Group. What was done well | – Ditto |
| What could be improved | – Ditto |

All suggestions need to be handled tactfully – 'It might be worthwhile trying to put that in a slightly different way and see how it works. Could we try something along the lines of.............' Suggestions and criticism are only acceptable when combined with positive alternative proposals.

If everyone is prepared to be taped and the group follows these rules scrupulously the threatening aspect is reduced to an acceptable level and a truly invaluable session usually results.

If you don't have access to a video, consider seeking help from an outsider for practice viva sessions. Trainers, current or past examiners and course organisers will usually be only too willing to help if they can. Often useful tips can be obtained from colleagues who have recently sat the examination and passed. The latter may also be a bit less intimidating!

## Handling the questions

With the first viva being based on the questionnaire the candidate immediately starts with an advantage. The material is under the candidate's control and with proper preparation that puts the direction the discussion takes into the candidate's hands. YOU ARE IN CHARGE.

Prepare thorough model answers for every aspect of the questionnaire. For example, every member of practice staff (attached and employed) should have their role clearly defined, and their training needs outlined. You should be able to explain who pays them and what difficulties they face in doing their job. Be prepared to describe what plans the practice has in this direction in the future, what is a contract of employment, who recommends the level of annual pay awards and so on. Talk to partners and the staff. Read about the business side of general practice and be prepared to quote the literature to justify your approaches and responses. You can only move up the examiners' marking sheet if you have prepared thoroughly by reading the material and then applying and quoting it.

The same approach should be adopted with regard to practice premises and equipment. It would not be reasonable to expect details of the finer points of the cost rent scheme but the broad concept and the pros and cons of practice-owned premises versus health centres might make the basis of an interesting discussion. There is very rarely only one correct answer. For each piece of practice equipment make sure you have a sensible rationale for its use in everyday situations. What are the advantages and disadvantages of having it in the practice? Think of practices and situations other than your own. Compare the needs of a rural practice with an urban one – a town GP with an active paramedic service might think a defibrillator unnecessary and refer all potential myocardial infarcts to hospital for consideration of thrombolytic therapy. On the other hand, in a rural practice this piece of equipment might be a valuable additional tool, particularly if the local charities have raised the money! Again, it should not

be beyond the wit of intelligent postgraduate students to find appropriate discussion articles in the literature.

The message is quite clear – IF YOU PUT IN THE QUESTIONNAIRE DETAILS OF STAFF, EQUIPMENT, PRACTICE ARRANGEMENTS, FUTURE PLANS, RECENT AUDIT OR CLINICAL PROBLEMS YOU MUST BE PROPERLY PREPARED TO TALK ABOUT EACH SUBJECT IN GENERAL TERMS AND SHOULD BE ABLE TO QUOTE THE LITERATURE TO SUPPORT YOUR DATA!

When it comes to the diary of patients, prepare a crib. A single file card for each patient should be clearly numbered and the pile of cards held soundly together with a treasury tag in the top corner. This will prevent the disaster of nervous hands dropping the cards in the heat of the moment and the viva disintegrating into something resembling a Tommy Cooper sketch as you struggle to get them off the floor and back into order. The briefest of details of the case are all that are required since the viva will involve the broader issues. Organised, common-sense protocols for the management of emergencies, common minor illnesses and chronic diseases are mandatory. Put the options, discuss the implications and make a choice – justifying it from the literature. Similarly, an organised, sensible prescribing policy with possible alternatives and an indication of cost implications is required. It sounds a tall order but as the reading and preparation progresses a structure emerges and can often result in an improved performance in one's day to day work. In reading about the log diary cases make a note of two or three papers from the literature for each patient. As the viva approaches commit these to memory and again use them to illustrate and justify your approach. Two or three sore throats, a couple of repeat prescriptions for the pill and a few blood pressure checks reduces the volume of memory required!

The problem solving viva will, surprisingly, test the candidate's ability to solve problems! As in the MEQ, you will be faced with dilemmas, conflict situations, hot topics and controversial subjects. The same skeletons that most find useful in the MEQ can also be brought into play here and a good selection of prepared starting phrases will give a few extra seconds of thinking time. Consider the options available to you, the implications of those options and make a choice, ideally justifying that approach from the literature. Then await the applause!

For example:

Examiner: A 66-year-old retired pharmacist comes to see you with a history of deteriorating vision for the last 4 months. What areas would you want to cover in your consultation with him?

Candidate: 'Well, there are obviously several aspects to be considered.' (Begins with a prepared starting phrase, and then selects a skeleton as an appropriate model to flesh out...)

'We would perhaps start with the patient's history of the problem and include in that particularly the patient's own ideas, concerns and indeed expectations. As a retired pharmacist the patient may have professional knowledge as well. This might be being considered appropriately by the patient or his ideas and knowledge may be out of date, incomplete or distorted by emotional involvement.

'Then I think I might need to examine the eyes, testing the visual acuity and with the ophthalmoscope have a look particularly for glaucoma and cataract as the likely treatable culprits. I might, as part of the examination, want to test the urine and take the blood pressure. If the pupil is small I might need to dilate it with a short acting mydriatic but I might need to consider how the patient was going to get home, for instance would he be fit to drive.

'Obviously I would want to explain to the patient in terms he understands the nature of the problem as far as possible at that stage. Depending on what is found we might agree that the most appropriate action is to do nothing. Or I might (with the patient's permission) write to the optician explaining our plan and perhaps involve him in follow-up examinations. We might agree that the most appropriate course of action is to refer to a consultant ophthalmologist. The latter might be an NHS or private referral depending on the patient's means and wishes.

'I read a review article recently concerning the ability of GPs to detect diabetic retinopathy on a single examination with an ophthalmoscope. The results were not terribly impressive and I would think that most GPs might err on the side of caution in this situation and lean towards the referral option, depending on what is found and the patient's wishes.

'Finally I would want to outline to the patient the referral process and how and when his appointment will be communicated to him and whatever action we have decided on it is likely we will have to consider follow up arrangements.'

Look at the marking sheet and decide at what level that answer could be marked. Reading the literature and practicing viva technique is all that is required to reach this standard.

# Oral questions

The following selection of oral questions is intended to serve two purposes. Firstly, it should give candidates preparing for the orals an idea of the type of questions that could be put to them. Secondly, it may serve as a bank of questions for study groups to use in mock vivas. Experience shows that the latter is invaluable preparation.

### Problem definition

1. You are called at 10.30 p.m. to see a 60-year-old man with a history of chest and epigastric pain for the past 2 hours. What areas would you wish to cover in this consultation?

2. A 70-year-old lady comes to see you and rather reluctantly admits to a 6 month history of intermittent spotting of blood per vaginum. Gentle examination reveals only the presence of atrophic vaginitis. Outline the plan for your consultation and further management from this point.

3. During evening surgery your receptionist asks you to see urgently a 55-year-old man who has been brought down to surgery by his wife. He last attended the surgery 10 years ago with a boil but was

found at home by his wife when she returned from her part time job that afternoon having suddenly become 'unwell'. He says he feels a bit weak, looks a little pale but otherwise thinks a lot of fuss is being made whereas his wife appears very anxious and on the verge of tears. Much to your surprise examination reveals a gross tachycardia, BP 100/60 and bilateral basal crepitations. An ECG shows a supraventricular tachycardia with a ventricular rate of 180/min. You advise immediate admission to hospital but this is dismissed by the patient who proposes to drive home. What do you do now?

4. A 38-year-old interior designer who you know has a highly successful business comes to see you requesting a letter. She has referred herself to a private clinic recognised as a national centre of excellence with a view to obtaining in vitro fertilisation but has been told that she cannot be seen without a referral from her general practitioner. She clearly regards this as bureaucracy gone mad and a waste of everyone's time – particularly hers. What would you do?

5. You are telephoned by the police and requested to attend urgently a 45-year-old man who is a patient of your partner. On arriving at his house you find him very disturbed, pacing the floor, pushing the furniture around and talking continuously, incongruously and loudly. He acknowledges your greeting by picking up a china figure and hurling it into the corner of the room. What factors do you take into account when handling this difficult situation?

6. Your receptionist receives a request from the husband of one of your patients for a home visit. His 25-year-old wife has been discharged 2 days ago after a miscarriage at 8 weeks. What is your response? What areas would you wish to cover in the consultation?

7. What is the value of self-help groups?

8. What are your indications for the admission of a patient to a hospice?

9. You visit a 65-year-old lady 2 weeks after the sudden death of her husband from a myocardial infarction. What would you wish to discuss with her? Do you routinely initiate further follow-up after this consultation? Why/Why not?

10. What problems might be faced by a newly diagnosed epileptic aged 16?

11. What problems might be faced by a newly diagnosed diabetic aged 76?

12. What problems are faced by a 64-year-old widow discharged from hospital to a Part III home following a left hemiplegia from which she has made a partial recovery?

13. 'She's getting too much for me with these falls – you'll have to put her in a home.' These are the opening remarks from a 50-year-old spinster who gave up her job 2 years ago to look after her frail and dementing mother now aged 80. How do you respond?

14. What is the role of a general practitioner in detecting children with impaired hearing? How might children with partial deafness be detected early? Why does this matter?

15. It is 11 p.m. and you are exhausted having seen 48 patients in surgery that day and done five calls during the evening for relatively minor problems. The telephone rings again about a 78-year-old resident of a local nursing home who has fallen out of bed. The patient apparently has pain from the top of her right leg and the nurse says 'Shall I call the ambulance or do you want to come and see her?' What would you reply?

16. The neighbours of a 90-year-old lady request your attendance at 2 a.m. The previous evening she has been burgled but fortunately only her purse containing loose change has been taken. Nevertheless she is understandably shaken and upset. Her neighbours expect you to 'give her something for the shock'. What could you do to help?

17. A 45-year-old lady comes to see you and bursts into tears before she is able to say anything. You then discover that her husband has been impotent for two years. He is a diabetic and a patient at another local surgery. She says he resolutely refuses to

discuss his problem with her and certainly not with anyone else. How can you help?

18. For the third time in half an hour your receptionist interrupts your surgery and you are already running 40 minutes behind time. She has a hysterical mother of a 3-year-old on the telephone. The child has fallen against a knife and the mother thinks the knife has 'gone right in her eye.' What do you do? This is the child's third episode of head trauma in the last 15 months. What issues does this raise?

## Management

1. You have just called the second patient of your Monday morning surgery into your consulting room when you are called urgently by your receptionist. An elderly man has collapsed in the main waiting room and is apparently unconscious. How do you respond?

2. A 24-year-old woman consults you on a Tuesday morning with slight frequency and dysuria which she has had for the previous 24 hours. She has not tried self medication. What would be your management? Would you have done anything differently if she had consulted you at 6 p.m. on Friday? What if she was departing for a holiday in Nepal in 48 hours?

3. A mother consults you about her child's first vaccinations which are due in 3 days' time. She has become increasingly worried about the pertussis vaccine. She thinks her sister had fits as a child but as she moved to Australia 6 years ago and has now lost touch with her she is unable to obtain details or confirmation. How could you manage this situation?

4. You receive a telephone call at home at 9 p.m. An 18-month-old girl has had a temperature that day and has suddenly become unrousable and started shaking. Describe your management.

5. One of your patients telephones for advice. She has just missed two periods and thinks she may be pregnant for the first time. She has not done a pregnancy test but is concerned because she has been in the house of a neighbour whose youngest child now may have german measles. How do you respond?

6. What are your criteria for diagnosing hypertensive?

7. What investigations would you pursue in a newly diagnosed hypertensive?

8. What would be your first, second and third line treatments for hypertensive?

9. How can you help a 56-year-old man who presents with what is clinically his third attack of gout in the last 6 months?

10. You receive an urgent message at 10 a.m. A mother has just found her 5-month-old baby apparently dead. Describe your management.

11. You are called out-of-hours to an 18-year-old with an exacerbation of his asthma. He is on no prophylactic medication and ran out of his Ventolin inhaler a few days ago. He has become increasingly short of breath and wheezy in the last 24 hours. He finds it difficult to talk in more than short sentences and his peak flow is 200 l/min. What would be your management?

12. You receive a note in the post from a teacher at a local primary school. One of your patients is in her class and is aged 7. He has told her that his step-father has been fondling his genitalia. The teacher has asked his mother to bring him to see you that afternoon but she has not indicated to the mother the reasons for the consultation being required. How would you handle this difficult situation?

13. Under what circumstances would you refer a patient with asthma to a consultant's out-patient clinic?

14. Why might you refer a patient with angina to a consultant's out-patient clinic?

15. A patient who is becoming increasingly disabled with emphysema requests a supply of domiciliary oxygen. How do you respond?

16. What is your management of a patient who presents with a sore throat of 4 days' duration?

17. You decide that a patient requires compulsory admission under the Mental Health Act. What sections are appropriate and how do you proceed?

18. A 56-year-old man comes to surgery with

a history of 6 weeks' flatulent dyspepsia aggravated by food and unrelieved by propriretary antacids. How would you handle this situation?

19. You receive a request to visit a newly registered patient at home. After arriving you discover that he is a Temazepam addict. He says he takes 150 mg per day and aggressively demands 4 weeks' supply. How would you handle this situation?

## Prevention

1. How do you achieve a high uptake of cervical cytology?
2. How would you organise your practice to increase the detection of cardiovascular risk factors?
3. Your senior partner suggests sending a written invitation to all patients aged 35–70 years for a blood pressure screening at a Saturday morning surgery. How do you respond?
4. A 45-year-old non-smoker requests combined oral contraception. What factors do you take into account when replying?
5. What do you know about the Forrest Report?
6. How would you improve record keeping in general practice in order to facilitate prevention?
7. What role do general practitioners have to play in helping patients give up smoking?
8. What are your criteria for screening patients for hypercholesterolaemia?
9. What are your criteria for starting treatment with lipid lowering drugs?
10. What is the value of a local child health surveillance programme?
11. What is the evidence for screening the elderly using the present arrangements detailed in the 1990 GP contract?
12. How could glaucoma be detected earlier? What are Wilson's criteria?
13. How do you detect problem drinkers?
14. A 16-year-old patient comes to see you for post-coital contraception. What areas would you wish to cover in this consultation?
15. An unmarried mother with two children under the age of 3 registers with the practice as a new patient. Neither of the chil-

dren has yet received any of the routine childhood vaccinations. How would you proceed with this consultation? Assuming consent for vaccinations is obtained, what forms and procedures will need to be completed and followed?

16. In the course of a routine consultation you notice that a 50-year-old married patient has never had a cervical smear. You raise the matter and in the ensuing discussion she says 'I've heard that you doctors only take smears to reach your targets so you can make more money. Isn't that true?" How do you respond?

17. A baby is diagnosed as being severely physically and mentally handicapped due to congenitally acquired rubella. What steps could the practice have taken to avoid this tragedy?

18. Why might a practice fail to achieve the higher target rates for childhood immunisations?

19. You have 5 minutes left of your 10 minute consultation with a 27-year-old woman. What aspect of preventative medicine would you wish to raise with her in this time? Justify your choice.

## Practice organisation

1. Your practice has decided that it wishes to expand its use of computers. Presently there is a single terminal used as a basic age-sex register, for repeat prescribing and as a partial morbidity register for asthma, diabetes and hypertension. The partners now wish to have terminals in every consulting room with a view to using the computers rather than manual records for all routine matters. You have been given the task of selecting the best computer system for the practice. How would you proceed?
2. What factors would you take into account when deciding whether your practice should or should not become fundholding?
3. What are the pros and cons of a practice using a deputising service out-of-hours?
4. What are the factors which produce an effective repeat prescribing system?
5. Your practice manager is retiring. The partners decide they would like to appoint a manager who would progressively under-

139

take a true management role rather than a senior administrative role. How would you go about making this challenging appointment?

6. What duties should a practice nurse undertake?

7. What are the pros and cons of working in a health centre owned by a third party?

8. What are the advantages and disadvantages of owning an ECG machine?

9. Your FHSA medical adviser has arranged to meet you and your partners. Your PACT data indicates that your prescribing is 30% more expensive than the regional average. How would you prepare for this meeting?

10. What is the role of the health visitor in the modern primary health care team?

11. Why do so few GPs undertake intrapartum obstetric care?

12. What are the advantages and disadvantages of the cost rent scheme? What is notional rent?

13. Your practice manager brings you figures which show the practice has experienced a 25% increase in night visits in the last 2 years. How would you react?

14. How do dispensing doctors receive their remuneration for the drugs they dispense?

15. How do non-dispensing doctors get reimbursed for drugs and vaccines they personally administer?

16. Your local diabetic consultant meets the practice to discuss his plans to discharge all of the non-insulin dependent and stable insulin using diabetics for follow-up in the practice diabetic clinic. You are aware that a recent audit of patients seen only in the practice has shown only 20% have had a fundoscopy in the last year. Indications from preliminary discussions from your practice nurse are that she sees no real problems with the current organisation and suggestions concerning change will be met with considerable resistance. How could you proceed?

17. One of your receptionists has been with the practice for 20 years. In the last month two of her colleagues have been to see you independently complaining about her authoritarian attitude to other members of staff. Last week one of your patients, who is also a personal friend, had a polite but firm word with you about his treatment by her when trying to book an appointment. This morning the practice manager has received a letter with similar content and tone. What are your options?

18. You are asked by your partners to prepare a plan to improve surgery security in order to protect doctors and staff from violent patients. How would you go about this?

## Communication

1. A 55-year-old woman asks for your advice concerning hormone replacement therapy. She had a natural menopause 5 years ago and has no significant past medical history or family history. What areas would you wish to discuss with her?

2. A 67-year-old former coal miner has been increasingly disabled over the last 2 years with chronic obstructive airways disease and pneumoconiosis. A recent prolonged exacerbation of his respiratory symptoms has led to your arranging a chest X-ray. Much to your surprise it shows a hilar mass which the radiologist comments is almost certainly an inoperable carcinoma of bronchus. He is coming to see you today for a review and the result of his X-ray. How would you proceed with this consultation?

3. The MacDonald children are well known to you. Aged 3, 5 and 8, hardly a week goes by without their mother bringing one or other of them to see you, usually with a minor self-limiting upper respiratory infection and often in 'extra/emergency' appointments. What factors might lead to this pattern of consulting? Is it appropriate? How might you attempt to change it?

4. What would you say to the mother of a 3-year-old who you have just diagnosed as having asthma?

5. A 41-year-old company director comes to see you. He has been suffering from epigastric pain and flatulence after food 'for a while'. A golfing partner lent him half a dozen omeprazole tablets at the weekend and his symptoms have now completely disappeared. Not surprisingly he requests a prescription from you for a further supply

so that he can give his friend back the ones he has borrowed and keep some for himself in case of further trouble. He is already rather irritated as he has tried to buy some at the chemist, was refused without explanation and he's 'far too busy to spend time messing about at the doctors'. What would you say to him?

6. A 43-year-old attends your practice nurse for a routine smear. The result is CIN III and you refer her for coloposcopy. It is 9 months before she attends the clinic where the diagnosis is confirmed and her abnormal epithelium is ablated by laser. A few days later she attends surgery seeking an explanation from you. The hospital told her she had the worst kind of precancerous lesion. 'Why did you not arrange for me to be seen urgently?' How would you reply?

7. You are consulted by a 23-year-old mother of 8-month-old twins. She normally sees your partner. Following her post-natal examination she started the progesterone-only pill but had to discontinue this because of persistent headaches. After several further consultations she and her partner decide to use the sheath for contraception. She is horrified to become pregnant within a few weeks. Further consultations follow and a referral is made requesting a termination of pregnancy. She is seen in the outpatients department by a registrar who agrees to arrange her admission for the termination. He also suggests she sue her GP since sheaths were an inappropriate method of contraception given the circumstances. She seeks your further advice and support in pursuing her case against your partner. What would you do?

8. A 48-year-old diabetic is referred to you by your practice nurse. Her control has been increasingly poor over the last 12 months despite apparent compliance with diet and maximum oral hypoglycaemic therapy. Her opening remarks are 'If I have to inject myself with insulin I would rather die.' How can you help her?

9. A 35-year-old man attends surgery. He has recently been treated with Beconase for rhinitis without benefit. His girlfriend is keen on alternative therapies and has read

that this can be caused by an allergy to beans, oranges and bananas. They come to see you requesting a referral to a distant hospital to see a consultant in clinical ecology. How would you respond?

10. A 34-year-old woman registers with you having moved into the area. In the next 3 months she attends at least twice each week with a variety of vague non-specific abdominal complaints which increase in number despite your best attempts at diagnosis (possibly irritable bowel, ?gynaecological), investigation (all normal) and symptomatic treatment. Her old notes then arrive from the FHSA which consist of four gusseted Lloyd-George envelopes detailing multiple symptoms, investigations and referrals for the past 8 years which have all failed to discover pathology or alleviate symptoms. How might your next consultation proceed?

11. A 19-year-old comes to see you asking to read his medical record envelope. What would you say?

12. You are called at 10 p.m. by friends of a 15-year-old who has taken 12 Paracetamol tablets 4 hours ago as a parasuicidal gesture. How would you handle this consultation?

13. A 20-year-old university student comes to see you requesting a termination of pregnancy. You confirm a 6 week pregnancy. She tells you that she has been in a stable relationship with her boyfriend for the last year and they have been having intercourse for the last 6 months, sometimes using a sheath and sometimes not. How would you respond to this request?

14. A couple in their 40s come to see you. The husband states their marriage is in difficulties and they need your help. He says his wife is not interested in sex. She seems reluctant to enter into a discussion. How might you help?

15. A 31-year-old woman comes to see you. She does not know where or who to turn to for help. For the last 2 years her husband has been drinking heavily, he lost his job a year ago and they are heavily in debt. What can you do?

16. A 21-year-old comes to see you as a temporary resident on a Saturday morning. He

states he is a registered drug addict on methadone and is visiting friends for the weekend. Unfortunately he has left his methadone at home and he now needs a supply to last until he returns home on Tuesday. How do you respond?

17. A 21-year-old chef comes to see you requesting a HIV test. How would you counsel him?

18. A 45-year-old lady consults you about a minor matter and then mentions that she was a victim of sexual abuse from her elder brother when a teenager. She still has regular nightmares and never married, having 'always been afraid of men' since. She has never discussed this with anyone before. How would you proceed?

## Professional values

1. A 23-year-old man comes to surgery having recently returned from a business trip to Thailand. He gives a history of a 5 day urethral discharge and clinically he has a gonococcal urethritis. You inform him of your provisional diagnosis and he replies 'I thought it might be. My wife must never find out about this – please don't write anything in my records.' How could you respond?

2. You see a 44-year-old man and give him a further 13 week certificate for back pain. He normally sees your partner and you note he has been unable to work for 2 years. All investigations have been negative and as far as you can see the therapeutic options have been exhausted. Later, after surgery, you are chatting with one of your receptionists who says 'By the way, I see that chap with the bad back was in again. He can't be too bad now – I saw him last week helping one of my neighbours rebuild his garden wall.' What would you do?

3. You have a 64-year-old man on your list with chronic renal failure. He is being treated by the regional centre of excellence with intermittent peritoneal dialysis and you hear little from him for some months. Then you receive a message from his wife. He has decided that his quality of life is such that he has had enough and wishes to

die. Consequently he is not going to continue with his dialysis. What would be your response?

4. A 15-year-old schoolgirl comes to see you bringing her older sister for moral support. She is 8 weeks pregnant and requests a referral to a gynaecologist in another town without her parents being informed. What would you do?

5. What patients might be booked for a GP maternity unit?

6. You see a patient for ante-natal booking. This is her second pregnancy and she has an unblemished past obstetric and medical history. She would like a home confinement and has marshalled her arguments well. The current practice policy is to refuse all requests for home confinements. How might you reconcile these dilemmas?

7. You have an epileptic who has two fits within 3 months. You then discover that despite advice documented in his records to inform the DVLC somehow he has retained his driving licence and continues to drive. What would you do?

8. A patient of yours requires a form completing to accompany her proposal for life assurance as part of her endowment mortgage. The insurance company informs you that she does not wish to see the report when completed before you post it to the company. One of the questions asked is 'Do you consider the patient to be at risk from HIV infection?' You note that 4 years ago before she moved to your practice she had a negative HIV test performed at her request following a break up of a heterosexual relationship. There are no other details and no identifiable lifestyle risk factors. How would you complete the form?

9. Should we ever perform an HIV test without the patient's consent?

10. A 45-year-old teacher from France registers with you as a patient. She is working here for a year on an exchange scheme. At your first consultation she produces a box of ampules which she explains her French GP gives her at this time every year to prevent winter colds. As far as you can tell from the enclosed data sheet (which is naturally in French) the ampules contain a mixture

of killed cell wall and microsomal extracts of common respiratory pathogens – allegedly providing passive immunological protection. Her first dose of this year's course is due today. What would you do?

11. A 22-year-old nurse asks you to remove all records relating to a recent termination of pregnancy. How could you respond?

12. An 18-year-old patient on your list attends for an examination to assess his suitability for the Army. You are both aware that a past history of asthma will disqualify him and that he had two mild episodes of wheezing apparently associated with respiratory tract infections 10 years ago with none subsequently. Examination findings are all normal and his peak flow is better than his predicted value. He asks you not to enter his past events on his form. Unemployment in his age group in your area is 30% and rising. What can you do in this situation?

13. You are consulted by a 24-year-old with high myopia. She has read about corrective surgery for myopia and is keen to have this. You know that a local consultant ophthalmologist is offering this service on the NHS but you also know that there is a waiting time of a year for cataract surgery. This is a cause of distress to a number of your elderly patients. How might you respond to this situation?

14. In response to requests from a number of patients your senior partner makes the suggestion at a practice meeting that you should run an additional surgery some evenings from 8 p.m. to 10 p.m. How might you respond?

15. You do an elderly driving medical requested by the insurance company on one of your patients. The findings are satisfactory and you present him with an account for the BMA recommended fee. He is surprised and objects, saying that he had the same examination last year with your partner who managed to perform the examination in 5 minutes instead of your 20 and didn't charge him anything. What do you do now?

16. Does fundholding present the medical profession with any ethical problems?

17. You receive an official complaint from the FHSA alleging that a newly appointed receptionist was overheard in a local shop discussing confidential medical details about a patient. What would you do?

18. In recent months the appointment system has been under constant pressure. Patients, receptionists and doctors are all having problems because of the non-availability of appointments for patients needing to see the doctor the same day but no one so far has had the time or the energy to suggest anything constructive. How might you approach this difficulty?

## Personal and professional growth

1. Why do you wish to join the Royal College of General Practitioners?

2. What are you going to be able to do for the RCGP?

3. What do you expect the RCGP to do for you?

4. You receive a complaint from the FHSA. You are happy that your handling of the case is exemplary but how will you feel? How might you cope with this pressure?

5. Morale in general practice is said to be lower now than for sometime past. What can you do personally so that you enjoy your work?

6. How are you going to stop yourself from burning out?

7. How are you going to keep up to date during the rest of your medical career?

8. What are the advantages of being a GP instead of entering another speciality or branch of the profession?

9. If you were Secretary of State for Health what would be the single most important thing you could do to improve the standard of patient care? Unfortunately, you have been unsuccessful in persuading the Treasury to increase your department's budget.

10. As a GP you receive on average 15–20 medical newspapers, magazines and journals each week. How do you handle this deluge of information so that you select the most useful and thus keep up to date?

11. Do you think paying GPs approximately £2000 per annum as a postgraduate education allowance is likely to encourage appro-

priate continuing medical education?

12. How will you try to ensure that your own continuing medical education will be appropriate to your needs?

13. What paper, article or book has had the greatest influence on your medical practice?

14. A favourite aunt has sent a friend £50 for passing the MRCGP examination on the condition that he spends it on a book relevant to general practice. What would you recommend? Why?

15. 'Research in general practice is best done by the university academic departments of general practice.' What do you think of this statement?

16. If you thought of an interesting research project to undertake in your practice where might you obtain help and advice?

17. Do you think general practitioners should have to undertake some form of assessment at intervals throughout their career in order to be reaccredited?

18. Some general practitioners undertake additional work as clinical assistants, in industry, become GP trainers, sit on the local medical committee and so on. Is this a good idea? Why?

# ■ Appendix

This appendix contains:

(i) Child Health Surveillance pre-certification form and details.

(ii) Cardio-Pulmonary Resuscitation pre-certification form and details.

(iii) The Practice Experience Questionnaire. These are self-explanatory.

(iv) An oral examiner's log.
This is filled in during the orals by the examiners to record the content of the viva. Note the requirement to try and cover the areas of competence across the sheet during the viva which may result in a sudden shift in the context and content of the viva questions.

(v) The examiner's marking sheet.
Note that it is not possible to score higher than 'Bare Pass' without justifying some approaches by reference to the literature of general practice.

N.M.

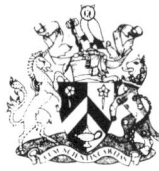

# THE ROYAL COLLEGE OF GENERAL PRACTITIONERS

## EXAMINATION FOR MEMBERSHIP

## CHILD HEALTH SURVEILLANCE

### Notes of guidance for candidates and assessors (March 1992)

All candidates presenting for the Membership examination in 1992 and thereafter are required to provide evidence of their competence in the practical aspects of child health surveillance (CHS) as a pre-entry requirement ot the examination. The other elements of the examination will continue to test knowledge, skills and attitudes appropriate to child health surveillance, as before.

### Certification

Attached is a form which, when completed by the assessor(s), will certify satisfactory proficiency in child health surveillance. A list of the surveillance tasks which must be demonstrated by the candidate is given on the reverse side of the Certificate. *No other form of certification will be acceptable.* The Certificate will remain valid for three years. Candidates resitting the examination within this period are not required to undertake a further test.

Each age group tested will require a separate signature since it is likely that these examinations will be carried out at different times and possibly in the presence of different assessors. If you do not live in the United Kingdom or the Republic of Ireland and perceive difficulty in completing the test by the closing date for the examination for which you are applying, please contact the Examination Department at the College for advice.

*The Certificate must accompany your application form for membership and the examination application fee.* Currently there are no exemptions from certification. Those who have been assessed in child health surveillance recently should have little difficulty in obtaining the requisite signatures on the Certificate supplied.

The Examination Departmant is unable to supply large quantities of certificates for the use of organisers of courses. However, it is permissible for copies of the Certificate to be made, provided that the most up-to-date version available is used for this and the Examination Department will be pleased to advise in this regard.

### Assessors

Certification can be carried out by:

(a)     Principals in general practice undertaking child health surveillance on a regular basis and approved to do so by the relevant FHSA or appropriate body.

(b)     other doctors, such as consultant community paediatricians and clinical medical officers, currently undertaking child health surveillance under the auspices of a local District Health Authority or appropriate body.

The Examination Board reserves the right to enquire into the credentials of those issuing Certificates as part of its policy of maintaining high standards in its assessment procedures. Enquiries are welcomed from those who might be uncertain of their position in regard to the certification of candidates.

Any expenses incurred are the responsibility of the candidate.

The College is grateful to those assessors who undertake testing on its behalf.

### Educational Courses

The Examination Board does not require candidates to have attended specific courses of training in child health surveillance prior to undertaking the test.

# ROYAL COLLEGE OF GENERAL PRACTITIONERS

## EXAMINATION FOR MEMBERSHIP

## CERTIFICATE OF COMPETENCE IN CHILD HEALTH SURVEILLANCE

CANDIDATE'S NAME: ................................................................................................

1    I have observed this doctor undertaking satisfactorily the examination of a child aged 6–8 weeks in each of the appropriate surveillance tasks listed overleaf.

Signature: ...........................................    Date: ...........................................

Name (Block Capitals please):    ...........................................

Address:    ...........................................

...........................................

...........................................

Professional Status ...................................    FHSA/Health Board/
Employing Authority ...........................................

2    I have observed this doctor undertaking satisfactorily the examination of a child aged 6–9 months in each of the appropriate surveillance tasks listed overleaf.

Signature: ...........................................    Date: ...........................................

Name (Block Capitals please):    ...........................................

Address:    ...........................................

...........................................

...........................................

Professional Status ...................................    FHSA/Health Board/
Employing Authority ...........................................

3    I have observed this doctor undertaking satisfactorily the examination of a child aged 36–48 months in each of the appropriate surveillance tasks noted overleaf.

Signature: ...........................................    Date: ...........................................

Name (Block Capitals please):    ...........................................

Address:    ...........................................

...........................................

...........................................

Professional Status ...................................    FHSA/Health Board/
Employing Authority ...........................................    147

*THIS CERTIFICATE REMAINS VALID FOR THREE YEARS FROM THE DATE OF THE LAST TEST*

| GENERAL | 6-8 WEEKS | 6-9 MONTHS | 36-48 MONTHS |
|---|---|---|---|
| 1. Seeks parents concern re: health, development and behaviour | | | |
| 2. Handling and approach to child | | | |
| 3. Makes adequate record | | | |
| **CHECK** | | | |
| 4. Weight | | | |
| 5. Length/ Height | ✗ | ✗ | |
| 6. Head Circumference | | | ✗ |
| **CHECK** | | | |
| 7. General behaviour | | | |
| 8. Appearance | | | |
| 9. Skin | | | |
| 10. Fontanelles | | | ✗ |
| 11. Palate | | ✗ | ✗ |
| 12. Motor tone | | | ✗ |
| 13. Reflexes | | ✗ | ✗ |
| 14. Co-ordination (fine motor) | ✗ | | |
| 15. Vision/ Eyes | | * | * |
| 16. Squint | | | |
| 17. Ears | | | |
| 18. Hearing | * | * | * |
| 19. Language/ Vocalisation | | | |
| 20. Heart | | ✗ | ✗ |
| 21. Femoral Arteries | | ✗ | ✗ |
| 22. Spine | | ✗ | ✗ |
| 23. Hips | | ✗ | ✗ |
| 24. Feet | | ✗ | ✗ |
| 25. Hernia | | ✗ | ✗ |
| 26. Testes | | ✗ | ✗ |
| 27. Genitalia | | ✗ | ✗ |
| 28. Bladder Control | ✗ | ✗ | * |
| 29. Bowel Control | ✗ | ✗ | * |
| **ADVICE RE:** | | | |
| 30. Health Education | | | |
| 31. Immunisation | | | |

* Check parents perceptions and refer if concerned. ✗ = not essential

Ref (i): Child Health Surveillance - A District Core Programme (BPA) 1990

(ii): Handbook of Preventive Care for Pre-School Children (GMSC/RCGP) 1988

(iii): Royal College of General Practitioners and British Paediatric Association - Guidelines for the training and accreditation of general practitioners - Child Health Surveillance, December 1989.

March 1992

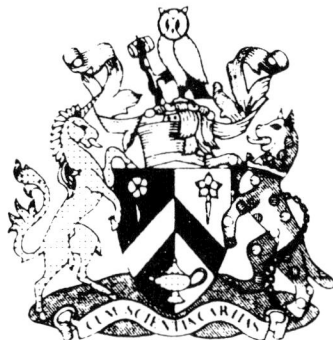

**ROYAL COLLEGE OF GENERAL PRACTITIONERS**

**EXAMINATION FOR MEMBERSHIP**

**CARDIO-PULMONARY RESUSCITATION (CPR) --- NOTES FOR CANDIDATES AND TESTERS**

---

All candidates applying to sit the MRCGP examination must provide evidence of competence in basic cardio-pulmonary resuscitation (CPR).

Certification

The certificate printed overleaf, which is based on the guidelines for basic life support issued by the Basic Life Support Working Party of the European Resuscitation Council in November 1992, when completed, will certify satisfactory performance in basic cardio-pulmonary resuscitation for the purposes of the examination. *No other form of certification will be acceptable.* The certificate will remain valid for three years. Candidates resitting the examination within this period are not required to undertake a further test.

The ideal performance of each activity and acceptable levels of variation are itemised on the certificate. The candidate must be able to achieve a pass in each activity but those who fail may be re-tested after instruction.

Candidates who do not live in the United Kingdom or the Republic of Ireland and perceive difficulty in completing the test by the closing date for applications are asked to contact the Examination Administrator for advice. **The Certificate issued must accompany the application form for Membership unless agreed otherwise**. If you are physically challenged and incapable of carrying out cardio-pulmonary resuscitation, please ask the tester to certify that you are competent in instructing a physically able person to perform CPR to the requisite level. A note should be made on the form if certification has been achieved in this way.

Testing

Many candidates will have access to hospital specialists in accident and emergency departments and anaesthetic departments. A certificate signed by a hospital consultant in the departments of accident and emergency and anaesthetics or by others with specific skills will be accepted. These could include general practitioners or doctors in HM Forces with a special interest and training officers in the Ambulance Service, Red Cross or St John Ambulance. The Examination Board reserves the right to enquire into the credentials of those issuing certificates as part of its policy of maintaining high standards in its assessment procedures. It welcomes enquiries from those who might be uncertain of their position in regard to the certification of a candidate. Alternatively the ambulance training/testing centres listed on the attached sheet are likely to offer local training and certification.

Any expenses incurred, including fees, are the responsibility of the candidate. We understand that there may be some variation in the charges levied for training and testing between centres because of local charging policies.

The College is grateful to those assessors who undertake testing on its behalf.

June 1993                                                                                  (test certificate overleaf)

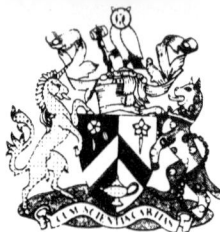

# THE ROYAL COLLEGE OF GENERAL PRACTITIONERS
## EXAMINATION FOR MEMBERSHIP

**CARDIO-PULMONARY RESUSCITATION PERFORMANCE TEST**
**Revised March 1993**
Candidates must obtain pass in each activity

Candidate's Name ——————————————— Date ———————

| Activity | Ideal Performance | Acceptable Variation | Pass | Fail |
|---|---|---|---|---|
| 1 Check for personal safety before treating the casualty Determine unresponsiveness | Shake by shoulders - ask loudly "are you alright?" | None | | |
| 2 Call for help | Call for help immediately | None | | |
| 3 Open airway and check mouth | Head tilt and chin lift | None | | |
| 4 Determine whether casualty is breathing or not | Look, listen and feel for breathing for 5 seconds | None | | |
| 5 Determine whether a pulse is present or not | Palpate carotid artery for 5 seconds | None | | |
| 6 Activate 999 system | ............. | None | | |
| 7 Initial ventilations | 2 slow ventilations Vol per ventilation 0.8 - 1.2 litres Inspiratory time per ventilation 2 seconds | 1 - 3 slow ventilations | | |
| 8 Cycles of chest compressions and ventilations | 15 chest compressions to a depth of 4 - 5 cms over the lower part of the sternum avoiding pressure on the abdomen or ribs. at least 70% correct ventilations at least 70% correct compressions Alternate 15 compressions at rate of 80 per minute with 2 ventilations. Vol per ventilation 0.8-1.2 litres. Inspiratory time per ventilation of 2 seconds. At least 4 cycles of compressions and ventilations must be performed. | Compression rate 60-100 per minute Average compression: Ventilation ratio over assessment period 15:2 | | |
| 9 Timing of activities | Step 1 to the completion of 4 cycles of compressions/ ventilations to be performed within 2 minutes. | Performed within 2 minutes 15 seconds | | |

Examiner's Signature _____   Result _____ Pass _____ Fail _____

Name _____   *Candidates who fail the test may be re-tested after instruction*

Address _____

150

ATTACH MANIKIN PERFORMANCE RECORD IF AVAILABLE
THIS CERTIFICATE REMAINS VALID FOR THREE YEARS FROM DATE OF THE TEST

# AMBULANCE SERVICE TRAINING/TESTING CENTRES

You are advised to contact the Chief Ambulance Officer or Training Officer at the locations listed below.

| | | |
|---|---|---|
| London | Bromley Training Centre<br>Crown Lane<br>Bromley | 081 464 7608 |
| | Heathrow Training Centre<br>Heathrow Airport Ambulance Centre<br>Building 450<br>Northern Perimeter Road<br>Hounslow<br>TW6 1JH | 081 759 3056 |
| | Ilford Training Centre<br>Auldborough Road South<br>Ilford | 081 983 8974 |
| | Fulham Training Centre<br>Fulham Ambulance Station<br>Seagrave Road<br>London<br>SW6 1RX | 071 381 4070 |
| Northern | Newcastle upon Tyne<br>Middlesbrough<br>Carlisle<br>Durham | 091 273 1212<br>0642 326316<br>0228 39441 x 45<br>091 386 4488 |
| Yorkshire | Bradford, W Yorkshire<br>Hull<br>York | 0274 651410<br>0482 561191<br>0904 628085/8 |
| Trent | Rotherham, S Yorkshire<br>Derbyshire<br>Leicestershire<br>Lincolnshire<br>Nottinghamshire | 0709 828820<br>0332 372441<br>0533 750700<br>0522 45171 x 27<br>0602 296151 |
| East Anglia | Cambridge<br>Norwich<br>Ipswich | 0223 411444<br>0603 424255<br>0473 49333 |
| North-west Thames | Bedford<br>Welwyn Garden City, Herts | 0234 270099<br>0707 327585 |
| North-east Thames | Chelmsford, Essex | 0245 443344 |
| South-east Thames | Eastbourne, E Sussex<br>Maidstone, Kent | 0323 21433<br>0622 747010 |
| South-west Thames | Banstead, Surrey<br>Worthing, W Sussex<br>London SE1 | 0737 353333<br>0903 691378<br>071 928 0333 |
| Wessex | Winchester<br>Ringwood<br>Isle of Wight<br>Chippenham<br>Guernsey<br>Jersey | 0962 60421<br>0202 896111<br>0983 528500<br>0249 443939<br>0481 25211<br>0534 59000 x 2329–2333 |

Oxford

| | |
|---|---|
| Wokingham, Berks | 0734 771200 |
| Deanshanger, Milton Keynes | 0908 262422 |
| Oxford | 0865 741841 |

South-western

| | |
|---|---|
| Bristol | 0272 277046 |
| Truro, Cornwall | 0872 78181 |
| Exeter | 0392 403339 |
| Gloucester | 0452 395050 |
| Taunton, Somerset | 0823 278114 |

West Midlands

| | |
|---|---|
| Dudley | 0384 455644 |
| Worcester | 0905 830630 |
| Shrewsbury | 0743 64061 |
| Stafford | 0785 61844 |
| Leamington Spa, Warwickshire | 0926 881331 |

Merseyside

| | |
|---|---|
| Liverpool | 051 260 5220 |
| Chester | 0244 362492/362632 |

North-western

| | |
|---|---|
| Manchester | 061 236 9456 |
| Preston | 0772 862667 |

SCOTLAND

| | |
|---|---|
| Paisley | 041 848 1434 |
| Ayr | 0292 284101 |
| Motherwell | 0698 64201 |
| Glasgow | 041 332 6001 |
| Edinburgh | 031 447 8746 |
| Aberdeen | 0224 681656 |
| Inverness | 0463 235789 |
| Dundee | 0382 816070 |

WALES

| | |
|---|---|
| Mold, Clwyd | 0352 700227 x 2123 |
| Caernarfon, Gwynedd | 0286 4811/2 x 126 |
| Caerleon, Gwent | 0633 421521 |
| Carmarthen, Dyfed | 0267 233232 |
| Brecon, Powys | 0874 711661 |
| Swansea | 0792 651501 x 227 |
| Pontypridd, Mid-Glam | 0433 217005 |
| Cardiff | 0222 552011 |
| Haverfordwest, Dyfed | 0437 767801 x 247 |

NORTHERN IRELAND

| | |
|---|---|
| Belfast | 0232 246113 |
| Antrim | 08494 67097 |
| Armagh | 0762 335121 |
| Londonderry | 0504 45171 |

REPUBLIC OF IRELAND

| | |
|---|---|
| Dr Gerard Bury<br>Department of General Practice<br>Royal College of Surgeons of Ireland<br>185 Harcourt Street, Dublin 2 | 0001 784422 |

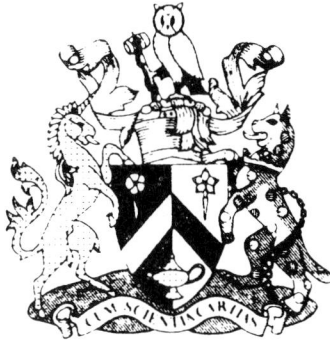

# THE ROYAL COLLEGE OF GENERAL PRACTITIONERS

# EXAMINATION FOR MEMBERSHIP

The oral examination will consist of two parts, each half-an-hour and each part being with a different pair of examiners.

The first oral will be devoted to examining the candidate using his/her Practice Experience Questionnaire as the basis for topics to consider. Although trainees and candidates from the Services may not have been able to influence the practices described, they will be expected to have a good working knowledge of the practice organisation, though not necessarily to justify it.

Part of the time will be spent on considering the practice, its facilities, organisation and services, and part on the clinical record. Candidates may bring to the examination brief clinical notes on the patients listed.

Candidates not in practice currently must complete the Clinical Diary and should describe a practice in which they have worked. If possible patients should have been managed recently in general practice, if necessary by undertaking some part-time or locum work.

The second oral will be based on topics arising from the presentation and management of clinical problems chosen by the examiners.

The candidate may also be asked to comment on issues relating to the profession in general and general practice in particular.

Candidates will be expected to satisfy the examiners that they can apply their knowledge and skills to total personal care in clinical, psychological and social terms.

Please note that there have been some alterations to the questionnaire (formerly called the Log Diary). There are partly to reflect the changes that have occured in practice organisation recently, or are expected to result from the 1990 Contract; and partly (as in Sections E and F) to make the questionnaire more relevant to the candidate's own learning and clinical experiences.

**The completed questionnaire should be returned to the Examination Department at the Royal College of General Practitioners, 14 Princes Gate, Hyde Park, London SW7 1PU.**

**March 1991**

# PRACTICE EXPERIENCE QUESTIONNAIRE (LOG DIARY)

The information requested in this questionnaire will provide a basis for discussion in the first oral. It will not, in itself, attract any marks.

## SECTION A. CANDIDATE'S PERSONAL DATA

1. Name:

2. Examination number

3. Address:

4. Your present status in general practice: (Please tick)

   Principal
   Assistant
   Trainee

5. Your total experience in general practice:

   Years
   Months

6. Length of time in present post:

   Years
   Months

## SECTION B. PRACTICE STRUCTURE

7. Total list size:

   Percentage of patients    Under 5          65–74          Over 75

8. Premises and Practice Features: (Please tick)

   Purpose-built                Urban
   Converted                    Rural
   Partnership-owned            Mixed
   Rented                       Dispensing
   LHA Health Centre            Budget-holding
   Other                        Undergraduate teaching
                                Training

9. Number of doctors providing General Medical Services:

   Partners full-time        Assistants
   Partners part-time        Trainees

10. Please comment on any special, social, ethnic or other features of the practice:

154

## SECTION C. PRACTICE ORGANISATION AND FACILITIES

11.     Staff. Please list the various categories of ancillary staff working in the practice and show the numbers in each category.

Nursing and Paramedical

| Employed | part/full |
|----------|-----------|
|          |           |

| Attached | part/full |
|----------|-----------|
|          |           |

Clerical and Administrative

| Employed | part/full |
|----------|-----------|
|          |           |

| Attached | part/full |
|----------|-----------|
|          |           |

12.     Is Child Heath Surveillance approved within the Practice?          Yes/No

13.     Is minor surgery approved within the practice?          Yes/No

14.     What health promotion clinics are approved within the practice?

15.     What additional clinics/ sessions exist within the practice?
eg obstetrics, immunisation, screening?

16.     What systems for audit exist within the practice?

17. What special diagnostic, therapeutic or other equipment is available within the Practice (eg ECG, sonicaid, autoclave)?

| Diagnostic | Therapeutic and other |
| --- | --- |
|  |  |

18. What diagnostic or therapeutic facilities are available by direct access outside the Practice (eg X-ray, ultrasound, endoscopy, physiotherapy)?

| Diagnostic | Therapeutic |
| --- | --- |
|  |  |

19. Is there a computer in the Practice?        Yes/No

If so, what are its principal uses?

20. How are out-of-hours duties covered?        (Please tick)

Rota within Practice                Rota with one other Practice
Deputising Service                Rota with several Practices

## SECTION D. WORK LOAD ANALYSIS

21. Please state the numbers of patients seen in a recent typical week.

a)    by all doctors

| | M | T | W | Th | F | S |
| --- | --- | --- | --- | --- | --- | --- |
| consulting am |  |  |  |  |  |  |
| consulting pm |  |  |  |  |  |  |
| special surgeries or clinics |  |  |  |  |  |  |
| new home visits |  |  |  |  |  |  |
| repeat home visits |  |  |  |  |  |  |

b)    by the candidate

| | | | | | | |
| --- | --- | --- | --- | --- | --- | --- |
| consulting am |  |  |  |  |  |  |
| consulting pm |  |  |  |  |  |  |
| special surgeries or clinics |  |  |  |  |  |  |
| new home visits |  |  |  |  |  |  |
| repeat home visits |  |  |  |  |  |  |

22. Does the Practice have acess to
a GP Obstetric Unit?　　　　　　　Yes/No

How many confinements were　　　　)　　　in complete care
there in a recent quarter?　　　　　　)　　　in shared care

23. What is the practice's consulting rate
(doctor-patient consultations per patient per year)?

## SECTION E. CANDIDATE'S OWN IDEAS AND LEARNING EXPERIENCE

24. Describe two or three features of the Practice which you have found to be interesting or stimulating; or which
have influenced your attitudes; or which have helped you improve your knowledge or skills; or an audit or study
that you have carried out.

25. What changes would you suggest for the next three years to improve the Practice?

## SECTION F. CLINICAL DIARY

Please list the relevant numbers of patients seen consecutively in each of the following categories: surgery attendances – 25 cases; home visits – 15 cases; out-of-hours emergencies – 10 cases including 2 night calls whenever possible. These cases will provide examples for examination of your clinical abilities. You may bring brief clinical notes about them to the examination.

| No. | Date | Patient's Initials | Age | Sex | Main reason for contact |
|-----|------|--------------------|-----|-----|-------------------------|
| Surgery Attendances | | | | | |
| 1. | | | | | |
| 2. | | | | | |
| 3. | | | | | |
| 4. | | | | | |
| 5. | | | | | |
| 6. | | | | | |
| 7. | | | | | |
| 8. | | | | | |
| 9. | | | | | |
| 10. | | | | | |
| 11. | | | | | |
| 12. | | | | | |
| 13. | | | | | |
| 14. | | | | | |
| 15. | | | | | |
| 16. | | | | | |
| 17. | | | | | |
| 18. | | | | | |
| 19. | | | | | |
| 20. | | | | | |
| 21. | | | | | |
| 22. | | | | | |
| 23. | | | | | |
| 24. | | | | | |
| 25. | | | | | |

| No. | Date | Patient's Initials | Age | Sex | Main reason for contact |
|-----|------|--------------------|-----|-----|-------------------------|
| Home Visits and repeat visits | | | | | |
| 26. | | | | | |
| 27. | | | | | |
| 28. | | | | | |
| 29. | | | | | |
| 30. | | | | | |
| 31. | | | | | |
| 32. | | | | | |
| 33. | | | | | |
| 34. | | | | | |
| 35. | | | | | |
| 36. | | | | | |
| 37. | | | | | |
| 38. | | | | | |
| 39. | | | | | |
| 40. | | | | | |

Out-of-hours and emergency calls. Indicate night visits "NV"

If sufficient cases in this category cannot be found please say why this is so.

| No. | Date | Patient's Initials | Age | Sex | Main reason for contact |
|-----|------|--------------------|-----|-----|-------------------------|
| 41. | | | | | |
| 42. | | | | | |
| 43. | | | | | |
| 44. | | | | | |
| 45. | | | | | |
| 46. | | | | | |
| 47. | | | | | |
| 48. | | | | | |
| 49. | | | | | |
| 50. | | | | | |

_____

_____

_____

_____

DATE: _____

**Please enter your names, examiner numbers and the date in the spaces provided above**

**MRCGP EXAMINATION – 293**
**Oral 2**

| Letter Code | Category | Examples of Justification | Category | Letter Code |
|---|---|---|---|---|
| O | *Outstanding* | A very rare candidate. Uniformly outstanding. Well-read, coherent, rational, consistent, critical. Without being asked, justifies approaches etc by reference to the literature. | *Outstanding* | O |
| E | *Excellent* | Extremely impressive candidate. Generally, as "O" – but not so uniformly well informed or perfect. | *Excellent* | E |
| G | *Good* | Generally impressive candidate. Well informed, coherent policies, fairly critical. Good decision making skills. Justifies majority of approaches well. | *Good* | G |
| S | *Satisfactory* | A candidate characterised by a reassuring solidness rather than impressiveness. Able to justify only some approaches well, but most appear sensible. Adequate, not good decision making skills. | *Satisfactory* | S |
| B | *Bare Pass* | Examiner is only just comfortable with candidate's adequacy. Not much justification of approaches, but important ones are sensible. Decision making and other skills tested are just, on balance, acceptable. | *Bare Pass* | B |
| N | *Not very good* | Questionable approaches, sometimes neither justifiable nor justified. Examiner is uncomfortable with candidate and his/her decision making skills, thinking him/her possibly risky in practice. Appears not good at applying basic knowledge. | *Not very good* | N |
| U | *Unsatisfactory* | Approaches are often inconsistent and rarely justified. Candidate does not appear capable of passing the exam overall. Poor at applying the knowledge base. | *Unsatisfactory* | U |
| P | *Poor* | Candidate clearly not passable, though slight evidence of ability. Generally incoherent approach to practice. No justification for specific approaches. | *Poor* | P |
| D | *Dangerous* | Candidate is worse than 'Poor': adopts such arbitrary approaches as to put patients at risk. | *Dangerous* | D |

**Please ring the letter code which best describes your impression of the candidate**

..........................................          ..........................................          ..............................

**Candidate**                                       **Candidate's Number**                              **Date**

1 [ ] (log diary)     2 [ ] (cases)          [ ]                                                       ..............................
**Which oral ?**                             **Trainee ?**                                              **Start time**

Please indicate by a tick which areas of competence were substantially explored within a topic. Then assign a mark for the topic. Do not try to cover every area within each topic — use the grid to guide your selection and use of subsequent topics.

| TOPIC | AREAS OF COMPETENCE | | | | | | | MARK | COMMENTS |
|---|---|---|---|---|---|---|---|---|---|
| | problem definition : | : management : | prevention : | practice organisation : | communication : | : professional values : | personal + profl. growth | | |
| .......................... | [ ] | [ ] | [ ] | [ ] | [ ] | [ ] | [ ] | .... | .......................... |
| .......................... | [ ] | [ ] | [ ] | [ ] | [ ] | [ ] | [ ] | .... | .......................... |
| .......................... | [ ] | [ ] | [ ] | [ ] | [ ] | [ ] | [ ] | .... | .......................... |
| .......................... | [ ] | [ ] | [ ] | [ ] | [ ] | [ ] | [ ] | .... | .......................... |
| .......................... | [ ] | [ ] | [ ] | [ ] | [ ] | [ ] | [ ] | .... | .......................... |
| .......................... | [ ] | [ ] | [ ] | [ ] | [ ] | [ ] | [ ] | .... | .......................... |
| .......................... | [ ] | [ ] | [ ] | [ ] | [ ] | [ ] | [ ] | .... | .......................... |
| .......................... | [ ] | [ ] | [ ] | [ ] | [ ] | [ ] | [ ] | .... | .......................... |
| .......................... | [ ] | [ ] | [ ] | [ ] | .[ ] | [ ] | [ ] | .... | .......................... |

**Safety ...**

If you are so concerned about this candidate's safety as to request a quartet, **tick [ ]** ⟶ **Why?** ..........................

..........................................................................................................................................

**Examiners' Names and numbers**

1 ..................................     no. .............     **Mark** ........

2 ..................................     no. .............     **Mark** ........

**Comments for possible feedback to Candidate**

..........................................................................................................................................
..........................................................................................................................................
..........................................................................................................................................
..........................................................................................................................................
..........................................................................................................................................
..........................................................................................................................................